Humming for Health:

Sound Tools for Physical and Emotional Balance

by

Kathleen Nagy
"The Sound Lady"

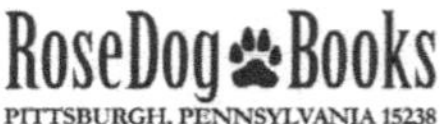

RoseDog Books
PITTSBURGH, PENNSYLVANIA 15238

The contents of this work, including, but not limited to, the accuracy of events, people, and places depicted; opinions expressed; permission to use previously published materials included; and any advice given or actions advocated are solely the responsibility of the author, who assumes all liability for said work and indemnifies the publisher against any claims stemming from publication of the work.

All Rights Reserved
Copyright © 2023 by Kathleen Nagy

No part of this book may be reproduced or transmitted, downloaded, distributed, reverse engineered, or stored in or introduced into any information storage and retrieval system, in any form or by any means, including photocopying and recording, whether electronic or mechanical, now known or hereinafter invented without permission in writing from the publisher.

RoseDog Books
585 Alpha Drive, Suite 103
Pittsburgh, PA 15238
Visit our website at www.rosedogbookstore.com

ISBN: 979-8-88729-124-6
eISBN: 979-8-88729-624-1

This book is dedicated to my mom.

Not a day went by without a song getting added to a
conversation, usually a lyric from a Broadway tune.
Her love of music is imprinted on my soul.

Thanks, Mom!

Table of Contents

Foreword

It is always good to know the biases of your authors and teachers. I figured that out as a student. The more I knew about the teacher, the more I could filter through their leanings and come to my own conclusions.

I am a musician. I come to this endeavor from the perspective of a sound master. My dominant sense for taking in and processing information is my hearing. Visually, I am not very interested in detail. Looking at something intensely is work for me, whereas listening to the fullness of the composites of a sound is a delight for me. I experience the world more through my ears than my eyes. That's just me. I like to play with sound.

This book is about listening to your inner wisdom, doing for yourself, and taking responsibility for your own innate healing abilities. In this book, you will find tools to discover how to use the sound of your voice to trigger your body's natural healing processes.

Throughout time, composers have sought after and attempted ascension upon the invisible wings of sound. For me, this sacred connection was remembered at the age of five on a Christmas morning when a toy trumpet sat calling to me from under the tree. I remember the tears of joy and recognition welling up from some deep and sacred place inside of me. Now, of course, it is comical and precious to consider my parents' bewilderment at this unexpected response to a plastic trumpet in a fake alligator skin case! But from that point on, I knew I was a musician.

I have several decades of professional experience as an orchestral musician. I majored in Music Education and Applied Music on French horn at Ithaca College and did my graduate work at Yale University majoring in French horn and minoring in Orchestral Conducting. I have taught music in both public and private schools from elementary school through adult education. I recorded a French horn solo CD called Prayer Songs, much of which I composed, performed, and recorded.

After 18 years of performing in symphony orchestras, playing the French horn, teaching music education, and directing musical theater productions, I was able to forage through the ingredients of crafted "classical" melody, harmony, and structure to find the power, beauty, and healing properties of tone and harmonics.

Now, for more than 20 years, I have been a BioAcoustic Research Associate, specializing in Voice Energy Analysis and Acoustic Biofeedback for sports or muscle injuries. I was a member of the Board of Directors for Sound Health International of Ohio from 2005 to 2009 and have worked closely with Sharry Edwards, founder of Human BioAcoustics – the study of the sounds made by humans.

After a lifetime of being surrounded by beautiful music and healing sounds, I created The Chakra SoundSpa Experience, a guided meditation mp3. This product teaches the listener to find the notes that vibrate their chakras. By vibrating the chakras with the voice or with the chimes meditation mp3, you can experience the unique sensation of tingling energy in your chakra centers while your emotions are calmed and balanced.

Humming your chakras with your voice is the most calming thing you can do for your emotions. Knowing your personal chakra scale defines the musical key of your body. The sound spectrum of our individual voices reveals the musical key to which our body's emotions are tuned. When our bodies hear and feel the vibrations that naturally resonate with our chakra energy centers, the result is almost instantaneous relaxation. Humming your personal chakra scale relieves anxiety, depression, and insomnia.

Women's health expert, Dr. Christiane Northrup, agrees in her book, *Women's Bodies, Women's Wisdom*, that, "Thankfully, you can own and operate your own state of health completely and fully by understanding the energy systems known as chakras." We will greatly build on this notion herein and explore how discovering your chakra scale is like finding the musical key to your body's emotional stability.

After spending 20 minutes listening to and humming along with your personal chakra chimes scale in the Chakra Sound-Spa Experience guided meditation, you feel as relaxed as if you just spent hundreds of dollars on a day at the spa!

By a leap of faith, I went from simply using sound to entertain people to being a believer in the power of sound to change the form and function of the body. When I played in orchestras, it was very much a team effort. Having to play perfectly in rhythm, perfectly in tune, perfectly balanced within the sound of the whole orchestra, not to mention being perfectly accurate playing all the notes in my part started to get old.

I noticed that older members of the orchestras who had played the old familiar pieces over and over again year after year were just sort of calling it in with a ho-hum attitude as if thinking, "Not this one again." One such piece was the 1812 Overture by Tchaikovsky. Living in Massachusetts and Connecticut, this piece was always the ending to a winter pops concert. It was also, of course, performed on the 4th of July and sometimes during a Christmas concert. It was as much a staple as Beethoven's 5th symphony.

One day, I decided that I did not want to be an older member of an orchestra that was just going through the motions. I knew intuitively that there was more to beautiful music than the ability to uplift spirits. I sensed a need to go deeper into the sound which I couldn't do in a group like an orchestra with all of its structure and mutual cooperation. I felt I was missing the forest for the trees. I knew I needed to step back and search within to satisfy my deep unspoken knowing about the powers of music and sound.

I remember the first time I sat with my horn in front of a music stand that had no music on it. It was scary and uncomfortable. I had been taught all my life how to properly interpret and perform the music of the classic composers with all their styles and nuances. Now, I was attempting to make my own sounds without playing a melody. I played single notes.

I sat in front of an empty music stand and listened to the sounds that were in me and wanting to come out. I had composed songs before, but this was different. I took a deep breath and put the horn to my lips. Sounds of birthing came out; egg-like sounds full of potential in their simplicity.

Simplify became my goal. Unlearning the complexities and focusing on the pure quality of the sound became my objectives. In this pursuit, I played with sound and the horn.

I would play a single tone and really listen to it. I wanted to experience it in my body and heart. I wanted to feel its power and vibration. There's an old tale about a farmer who played the fiddle. He'd play every night at the end of the long day of working on the farm. His wife listened every night hoping to hear him play something new or different.

She wondered why he just kept playing the same note over and over again. One night she went into the room where he practiced and asked him, "Why do you only play the same note over and over again? Why can't you play a jig or a melody like other fiddlers?" He looked at her, smiled, and replied "They just haven't found their note yet."

There I was, looking for my note.

The other experience that led me to believe that I could do more than entertain people with music was a picture that my wife took of me in a campground one evening after dinner. She was cleaning up and I took out my horn to play for a while. While I was playing, she looked at me with her aura-seeing eyes and said, "I wish you could see yourself the way I see you."

"What do you mean?" I asked.

"There are nature spirits flying around you, dancing to your horn music," she said.

I smiled and kept playing. She picked up a camera, said a little prayer that the camera would capture the spirits, and took my picture. When I saw the picture that the Instamatic camera had developed, I began to believe that I could do so much more with music.

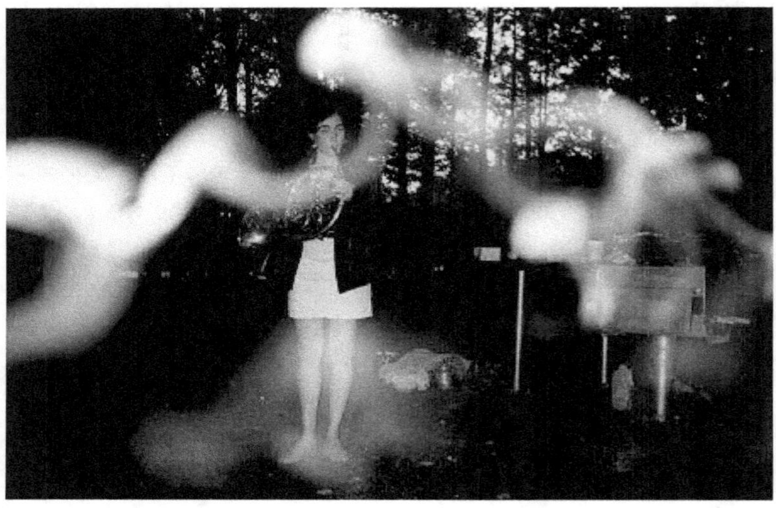

Another precursor to choosing sound and healing over music and entertainment was my first Sound Healing Conference in the late 1990's. Sharry Edwards was teaching. We had just learned that the frequency of white light was in between the notes B and C. I decided to do a white light meditation during a break in the conference and invited all the participants to attend. I don't have a picture of what happened, but it was such a powerful experience for many of the people there that they remember it more than 20 years later.

After hearing from them how it had affected different members of the circle, I realized I needed to start my next musical career playing healing sounds. Here is an excerpt from one member, Kathy Fucetola, who wrote about it in an email to me. "Floating with Sound," she called it:

"Kathleen is a professional musician. She plays a very mellow French Horn, one of my favorite instruments. She waited for us to settle in and then handed a crystal bowl to Lita. Someone somewhere was playing a soft drum. Lita began to spin sound out of the bowl and then it happened – Kathleen began to play her horn and the mixture of sounds was beyond sublime. Everything around us began to fade to nothingness and those sounds were all that was left. I have had what are called "Out of Body Experiences." As the sounds intensified and diminished, I felt myself lifting and then hovering above the group, the harmonics keeping me afloat. I could see those below me, eyes closed, lost to the spell of the music. It was over much too quickly, and I found myself back inside my body, back within that very quiet group anesthetized by the blend of sounds. There was applause and then everyone went quietly to their rooms, likely to deeply dream a repeat of the program. It should have been much longer. It should have been recorded."

Chapter 1

Listening

Receiving a Sound

Music shaped me into a natural listener. Listening is fun for me. For folks who are naturally visual, listening can be a chore. For me, the best way to really hear something is to be absolutely still. Picture a deer in the forest calmly grazing on some tasty grass, and when it hears something, the deer becomes still, motionless, and its ears are the only thing moving as they scan the area for predators. That type of alert stillness, that statuesque posture, is naturally conducive to listening.

Add to this:

1. An open and receptive mindset with the intention to receive
2. The patience to wait to hear it
3. The willingness and the courage to trust what you hear

The combination of these ingredients is optimal to quiet the mind and open the heart. This puts us in a receptive state. Getting quiet is the easy part. Having the patience to hear what you are asking to hear and then having the courage to trust what you hear and act on it is the hard part. Sometimes after stating an intention and being open to receiving, the answer doesn't manifest immediately. This is where patience comes in. I like to add to my intentions that what I am looking for should be for my highest good and the highest good of everyone else on the planet. That kind of ask usually takes a lot longer to manifest as the universe has a lot of coordinating to do!

There is a natural rhythm to things. True, we can use the power of our will to make something happen before its natural time, but the results are not always lasting. So, putting it out there in the etheric dimension also requires trust. Trust that the universe is acting on your behalf even if you can't yet see it.

Trust and patience are usually acquired talents. Older folks who have a history of seeing their questions and needs answered tend to have more patience with the process as their lived history provides a track record of their successes.

When I was living in Santa Fe, New Mexico, I met author, Nina Brown, at a networking lunch. There was a group in Santa Fe called Friday Networking Lunch. To join, we paid a yearly fee. Every Thursday we received an email telling us who we were having lunch with on Friday and what restaurant we would be meeting at. There were usually 3-6 people at the lunch, and it was a great way to meet new people who were also trying to market their businesses.

After the meeting where Nina came to speak with our small group, she and I had a chat while walking to our cars. She was organizing a weekend conference to promote her new book, *STAR – A Now State of Being*. STAR stands for Surrender, Trust, Allow, Receive. These were all things that I was doing daily. I told her I wanted to go to the conference but didn't have the money at this time. Nina told me that on the new Earth, money will not be the currency as it will be replaced by LOVE. She told me that what she had just learned about me during lunch was that I will be fine and not to worry.

As we talked, she realized that she had rented all the audio and video equipment for the conference but had forgotten to hire someone to run it all. I told her I could do that for her, and we made an agreement that I would do the work for the amount of the cost of attending the weekend conference. That was just one of the many examples of how things seemed to magically come together in Santa Fe. Surrendering to what is, Trusting that your God has your back, allowing for new information to appear, and being ready to receive it were all skills that I honed during my time in Santa Fe. It isn't called the Land of Enchantment for nothing!

Getting quiet was the easy part for me as I really enjoyed meditation exercises that quieted the mind. Practicing... every musician understands the long term benefits of practice. Meditations created a space where I could hear more. When my mind was not chattering away, I could expand my hearing range. With practice, I could listen for answers to prayers.

I could hear that still small voice inside, the inner guiding voice of intuition. Sometimes it is not received as a thought, but just a vague feeling. Nonetheless, it is all about being receptive and willing to expand your listening range.

I had often heard sounds in my ears throughout my life, but I mostly didn't pay attention to them. I didn't start listening to these sounds until I learned from Sharry Edwards, a pioneer in Human BioAcoustics, that these sounds are called Spontaneous Otto Acoustic Emissions (SOAE). They are made by the brain and the ear. The cochlea produces these sounds in an attempt to balance something that is out of balance.

Basically, it is a natural bodily process of using frequency to balance something in the body.

If you occasionally hear a high-pitched sound in your ear or ears that is there for a while and then is gone, that is an SOAE. If you can bring that sound down into a singing range, and then hum that sound, you will be increasing the energy of that sound far beyond what the cochlea can achieve by itself. If the sound in your ears is an SOAE, it will stop when it has accomplished its purpose. This is the best example of how the body and brain already use sound all the time to keep the body in homeostasis. SOAE's are part of a type of feedback system between the brain, voice, and ear. When we hear them, we can increase their energy and productivity by LISTENING to them and humming along.

Dorinne Davis has written extensively about the Voice Ear Brain connection. She is the authority on this subject. As an audiologist, she expanded the Tomatis protocols and understandings of how we process sound. She has written several books on the subject of the voice ear brain connection from her perspective. She has developed a protocol for assessing where the disconnect is and what type of therapy will reconnect it. Dorinne has developed a tool to reconnect the voice and the ear that sends the vibrations of your voice right into your ear.

What is listening but RECEIVING a SOUND?
Listening can also be receiving a thought.

Mostly, listening requires a mindset of willingness and receptivity. It requires a still mind. It is thought of as a "feminine" trait or Yin in Chinese medicine. Being a curious person also helps because you are more likely to listen to something that piques your interest.

Listening to motivational speakers on inspirational subjects can help set your mood and get you into a more positive mindset. Listening to quiet music can put you in a more receptive mood. Sometimes listening to music in a minor key, especially, is very helpful. Minor keys have a mournful tone that is conducive to deep thought. One of my favorites for this is Dvorak's G minor Symphony.

There are listening exercises where you focus your hearing on a sound coming from inside of your body to a sound in the room you are in. Then listen to a sound outside of the building you are in, then reverse back inside and repeat. If that is a chore for you, try listening to your favorite song and picking out the bass line, the guitar, the drums, or the keyboard instead of focusing on the words and melody. This might be more fun for you. Or try listening for the rhythm patterns and decipher whether the phrases of the song grouped in beats of two or three.

When I play harmonics as a meditation, I ask my brain to identify all the notes that are playing simultaneously. That is an overwhelming request for the brain, so it shuts down. Then I can just be inside the sounds. Not only is that fun for me, but it is also beneficial to my health because those sounds boost my immune system so that I rarely get sick. It also keeps my chops (mouth muscles) toned and it strengthens my lungs and pleases my ears. My point is, it will be most valuable to your health if you can find a way to make it fun and unique to you.

Having a quiet mind makes you a better listener. From this state, you are able to set a clear intention for your meditative practice.

Intention is simply a way of setting a goal. Yes, Spirit can read our minds without our even having to speak. But speaking an intention aloud is how to manifest it in this 3rd-dimensional Earth plane of zip code reality. Speaking a thought or sound makes it tangible. The thought is no longer invisible and silent. Speaking it gives it substance and body. It takes up space and exists.

Creation stories throughout ancient traditions, including Christianity, identify sound as the primal creative force. God did not just think, "Let there be light." God SAID it. It was the saying of it. The vibration made it manifest. When going into a meditative or prayerful state, it is best to speak your intention for that time out loud.

Then once you have set your intention begin to connect with your breath. Breath is also something we receive. I like to think of receiving a breath instead of taking a breath. There are many books written about the health benefits of conscious breathing. While I am not an expert in the realm of breathing, I have had a good deal of experience working with the breath. As an orchestral musician playing the French horn, I had to master breath management. There were some phrases that needed to be played in one breath. In order to play all those notes at the proper speed and volume, I had to know how to control the air coming into my lungs and the amount of air/sound going out of my lungs. In order to use your voice as a sound energy enhancement tool, you need to have sufficient breath to project and sustain the sound long enough for it to be effective.

In order to have this control over the breath, you need to engage the diaphragm muscle. Deep diaphragmatic breathing requires a deep breath. Let's look at the mechanics of breathing.

The best way to receive a deep breath quickly is to use a system we are already familiar with – a yawn. A yawn is the body's way of taking in air quickly because oxygen is needed. So, to simulate a yawn:

Open your mouth wide.
Open the back of your throat.
Lower the back of our tongue.

This will allow you to take in a lot of air quickly. As you simulate a yawn with your throat, relax your abdomen so that air fills your lungs. The rounded top of your diaphragm muscle will flatten downward to make room for the lungs to expand with air. As you exhale, you can use the diaphragm muscle to control the volume and speed with which the air is exhaled up and out of the lungs.

That exchange of oxygen and carbon dioxide within our cells is connected to the plant kingdom's exchange of carbon dioxide and oxygen. It is also connected to the breathing cycle of the Earth as She inhales Spring, holds in Summer, and exhales Autumn into the empty stillness of Winter. We are One Breath, in different rhythms and octaves. Receiving and releasing the pulse of life. The Breath is the pulse of life, and it moves like an infinity wave. I met the consciousness of The Breath one day at the end of an exhale. It was in that still place between in and out.

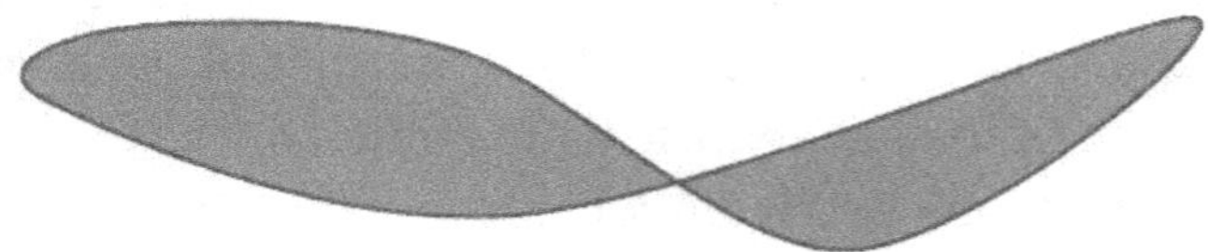

My friend, Jim, a mystical being, told me that "I AM the light of the Breath" and "I AM the light of the Transfiguration" hang out in the same frequency space in the ethers. I was intrigued as I never considered that there was a consciousness maintaining the in and out of breathing. I decided to build a relationship with "I AM the light of the Breath." I formed an intention to connect with IT.

Every morning, I would create these harmonic chords by playing a note on the horn and singing another note at the same time. The harmonic chords that I played correlated to specific organs and systems of my body; I would try to extend the duration of the chords as long as I could so the harmonics had a chance to grow and sound. This required great breath control.

While I was concentrating on the breath, I took the opportunity to create a relationship with IT. I began to talk to "I AM the light of the Breath" while I played these harmonics. I told "I AM the light of the Breath" that IT was the initiator of the sound. I explained to IT that the exhaled air vibrated the lips which creates the sound that traveled through the horn.

Jim explained that he sees the breath energy pattern as an infinity wave, a two-way street. We exchange energy with "I AM the light of the Breath" when our energy goes out into the ethers as an exhalation, and "I AM the light of the Breath" sends back the inhalation response from the other end of the infinity wave. This is the pulse of life. Later in this book, we'll discover what Jim calls "The Breath Pulse" meditation.

What is death but a final exhale not followed by an inhale?

In my own meditation, I included the awareness that "I AM the light of the Breath" and I were working together to create these harmonic chords. "I AM the light of the Breath" provided the exhaling impulse that vibrated my lips and carried the sound and my intention out into the world.

Jim came to visit about six months after I began consciously connecting with "I AM the light of the Breath." Daily, I thanked "I AM the light of the Breath" for each chord I had created with its help. I had not said anything to Jim about my budding relationship with "I AM the light of the Breath." One afternoon, after Jim had been meditating in my music/practice/meditation room, he came out and told me that I had taught "I AM the light of the Breath" that it initiated the sound of the notes that went into the horn and the sound of my voice as it vibrated my vocal cords.

He told me that "I AM the light of the Breath" was very grateful for this exchange of knowledge.

That's amazing!

I had actually accomplished what I had intended but given that I had no feedback in terms of language or intuition from "I AM the light of the Breath," I was very happy to hear Jim's confirmation from his discussion with "I AM the light of the Breath." Working with the consciousness of The Breath, using intention, and creating health-enhancing harmonic chords became a powerful and fun daily practice for me.

To help you find what works for you, here are a few stop-the-brain techniques that use the breath and worked for me.

1. **Release thought through the eyes**

   Inhale deeply, exhale letting your shoulders and lungs drop. Stay a moment in that still place before you inhale.

   Inhale the stillness while your eyes are closed. Exhale al the busy thinking out of your open eyes.

   Repeat until you have reached a calm and peaceful place of a quiet mind.

2. **"Always Here" meditation**

   Your "Always Here" is your higher self, the pure energy part of you that lives in the present moment and can access the answers to all of your questions. It is the part of you that lives on after you die. You are never separate from it, but you must be still and aware of the moment to access its wisdom. When you connect with it, you feel a deep peace and complete safety that knows no fear.

Ask a question on the inhale, answer it on the exhale.

Inhale and ask, "Always?"
Exhale answering, "Here."
Repeat several times then change the question
and answer.

Inhale asking, "Here?"
Exhale answering, "Always."
Repeat several times then change the sequence.

Inhale asking, "Always?"
Exhale answering, "Always."
Inhale asking, "Here?"
Exhale answering, "Here."
Repeat several times then change the sequence.

Inhale asking, "Always?"
Exhale answering, "Here."
Inhale asking, "Here?"
Exhale answering, "Always."

Repeat until you are in a state of oneness with your
higher self, completely relaxed, and at peace in the
present moment.

3. **Breathing and grounding meditation exercise**

Receive a breath through your nose and hold it in
your lungs while being aware of the exchange of
energy that is taking place.

Exhale silently through the mouth on a "ha" sound.
Repeat three times.

Receive a breath through the nose on the inhale, hold it in the lungs, and hug it gratefully with your ribs.

Exhale the love and gratitude carried on the breath with an audible "ha" sound.

Repeat three times.

Receive the air and consciousness of The Breath through your nose and hold it in your lungs.

Forcefully exhale on the sound of "uh" letting the shoulders drop and sending the energy into the Earth.

Repeat three times.

Inhale up from the Earth the love and support carried on The Breath and breathe it up the spine.

Exhale out the top of your head while envisioning a golden light, sparkling waterfall shooting out from your crown chakra and back down to Earth to complete the circuit.
Inhale up from the Earth up to your heart and exhale on a "ha" sound out of the heart chakra.
Sit in this space that you have created and enjoy!

Chapter 2

How to Hear Your Soul Sound
Advanced Listening

It was about 20 years ago now that I first heard my soul name. Imagine my surprise to be addressed by my guides as, "She Who Sings the Song of Source." I heard them say I sang from mountaintops and across vast expansive landscapes and that the song in my heart was the sound of the heart of matter, the sound of the heart of Spirit. They had heard me, loud and clear.

At the time, I only had a hint of the significance of hearing myself addressed in that way. Over the years, it gradually sunk into my consciousness and the knowledge of that vibration sustained me through very difficult times. It gave me context and purpose for the myriad of decisions large and small that kept me on my path of awakening.

What is your Soul Sound?

My understanding comes from the perspective of Source Sound Energy.

We are vibrational expressions of the Infinite Eternal that is becoming aware of itself within the heart of matter.

We are vibration. We are a symphony of frequency. We are Music!

Every cell in our body, and there are trillions of them, each one emits frequency and receives frequency. For the most part, harmony equals health, and dissonance equals dis-ease. Dissonance is not always unhealthy. There is a certain amount of dissonance that is necessary to counterbalance the harmony. The proper amount of dissonance allows us to stretch without breaking. It establishes a healthy amount of tension with our muscles, tendons, ligaments, blood vessels, capillaries, and all the tissues of our body.

Balance is the key. Certain activities require more tension, like a strenuous workout, but all tension seeks balance in relaxation and harmony. A healthy life is one that can handle the transition from tension to harmony with grace. Though we are always engaged in this dance of movement and vibration which can unbalance us at times, knowing your soul sound can bring you back to center.

The *source essence* of you is contained within a frequency – a speed of vibration. Your *source essence* is molecules of potential that vibrate at a certain number of cycles per second and create a form that is you in your Earth Body.

The source essence of you is contained within your soul's note or soul name.

Our soul name or soul sound is the essence of our souls. It is Our Source Sound, our Divine Alignment Sound. It connects us with our source essence.

Just like your Earth Body name, the more often you hear it spoken, the more easily you acclimate to your Earth Body. New parents repeat the names of their newborn children over and over again to them. As children, we hear our name and begin to identify with it. We begin to pay attention when we hear our names from our parents. Our heads turn to them as they speak it. The more they say our name, the more we identify with it. In the very same way, the more time you spend going within to hear your soul name, the stronger the connection becomes.

We have the opportunity to remember our soul name, our universal identity, prior to taking on this Earth Body. It is the remembering to resonate with the essence of your immortal, eternal soul, that helps solidify your new 5th-dimensional consciousness.

The sound of the words of your soul name contains the essence or source energy of your soul. Your soul's original expression, its original intention.

This concept of Source Sound is all part of a *Universal Language of Frequency*. Most of us have forgotten it, some of us are remembering it. Music is said to be the universal language here on planet Earth. Frequency is the language of the universe. Everything is math, and we are all part of a mathematical matrix.

In the *Universal Language of Frequency*, the fundamental tone is "ONE." This tone of **One Life** fills the universe, AND the Tone of the Universal One Life is filled with the purpose and reality of Unity and Love.

Some sounds can be symbolic. A fundamental understanding in ancient Chinese is the Wu Chi, the Om, the ALL. It is Sacred sound; it is not a particular pitch, but it is in everything and every dimension, for it is the space in between matter. All tone tends to seek resolution in the fundamental. It is the place to which all sound returns.

Within the One Tone of Life filled with the purpose and reality of Unity and Love, you – your frequency – is part of all of it. Your frequency is one of those intentions, hopes, and desires expressed by the One Life, the One Love Tone.

Your source sound, note, or name is part of the ONE LIFE LOVE TONE.

Understand that sound itself is neutral. It is just a carrier wave, a cable, a string as in string theory; sound is a vehicle for the transportation of energy. So your source energy is carried on a sound wave full of the intention of you. The intentions, hopes, and desires contained in the release from THE Source Energy, from Source Energy which desires to become aware of itself within the heart of matter with great love, released the thought of you and the intention of you within a sound.

Just like the creation story in the Bible, in the beginning was the WORD. The WORD is the sound of THE Source Energy, and the Word was made flesh. Source vibrated and created matter.

Your soul's essence is a sound, a word, or phrase expressed by THE SOURCE in a desire to become aware of your aspect of itself within the heart of matter.

This thought alone is very comforting, and there are many great possibilities for using the knowledge of your soul sound, name, or note.

Benefits of resonating with the knowing of your soul's essence within the fundamental ONE sound include:

1. Redefined sense of purpose.

    In those times when we are lacking motivation or stuck in a non- productive pattern, saying our soul name or humming our soul note can take us into a different, more productive mindset.

2. More efficient use of your energy.

    When we are not operating from our true self, when

we are just going through the motions, checking items off our to-do lists, we may feel like we are accomplishing things, BUT from our soul's perspective, we are wasting energy. We are giving energy to and creating things that do not feed our soul's purpose. Our soul's hopes and dreams are not being met. Our life is a continuum of events that attempt to steer us back to our path. Our soul's purpose can be understood when we know who we truly are. We are Loving, gifted, unique vibrations with things to offer that only we alone on Earth can do. When we know our soul sound, soul name, or soul note, our path becomes much clearer.

3. A re-found LOVE of yourself.

    There is nothing like the experience of realizing the great love that is in us or the enormous love that we are capable of giving and sharing when we are doing what we came here to do. Chanting our soul sound is one of the most affirming things we can do for ourselves. It sets up a field of well-being that changes everything. Sitting inside of this sound vibrates us to our very souls and gives us energy.

4. Making better decisions.

    We are always making decisions about how to use our time, whether we should do this or that, go to this event, take this job, move to this new home, pursue this relationship? Remembering our soul's purpose quickly redirects us down the right path and helps us make a decision that we won't later regret. Knowing your sacred sound is empowering in so many ways. The more you are aware of it and spend time inside of it, the more it creates sound wave connections that weave the matrix of your consciousness with your souls' purpose. This solidifies you and your Earth Body as a viable container, receiver, and transmitter of your soul.

THAT IS WHY WE ARE HERE. To receive, transmit, and store LOVE.

How to Listen and Hear your Soul Sound

Learning to hear your soul sound is an advanced listening skill. As a symphonic musician for 20 years, I honed my listening skills by knowing my part of the score and how the music in front of me meshed with the music of all the other instruments. I have spent a lifetime enveloped in sound. As a musician, band director, choral director, music teacher, sound healer, and voice energy analysis practitioner, I have spent a lifetime listening to and being surrounded by sound.

Hearing your soul sound is an advanced listening skill.

How well do you really listen and hear? How often are you still enough to really hear? Are we really listening to what others are saying and hearing their intentions? Or are we interrupting others to quickly express our opinion?

Listening and hearing are very feminine, very receptive. Listening is a skill that can be developed with practice. Make a new habit of really listening and hearing the thoughts and intentions of people, places, and things. Use all of your senses to really hear it, but use your senses from a space of connection with your heart. Let all of your senses be filtered through your unconditional heart center so that they can be informed within the context of unconditional love.

"Hear" is a large part of the word heart. Listen with your heart. Sit in a still, quiet space. Listen for your sound. Does the space created by the sound have a color, a word or phrase, a scent, or a feeling that is apparent to you? Hear with your heart your soul's essence within this 10-note melody.

C   E   F   F#   D   E♭   B♭   E   B♭   C

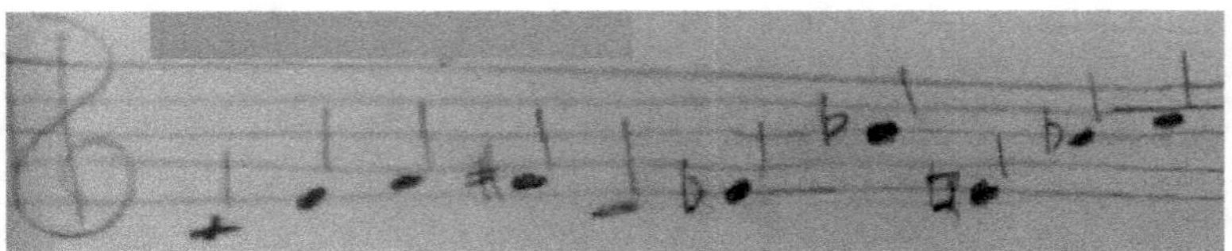

When this ten-note melody of the Universal language of Frequency was downloaded to me, I scribbled it down immediately. These sounds create a space that resonates with human beings who are remembering their expansive, unconditional loving selves.

Feel the quality of energy change in the room as you play it.

Listen for your soul name. Let it float to you carried on the sound waves of your heart as they connect with your source essence. **Hearing your soul sound is an advanced listening skill that can be developed with practice.**

Chapter 3

Matter Vibrates, Sound is Vibration

Sound Affects Matter

Since we know that matter vibrates, and we know that sound is vibration, it is logical to deduct that sound affects matter. You just need to **know the right sound for the right piece of matter.**

I'm sure you have seen those videos of an empty wine glass being shattered into a million pieces while sound was being blasted at it. Sound can destroy matter and sound can repair matter as you will see in my aura camera case study.

I understand that using sound to repair matter is out of the frame of reference for most people. If most human beings have an ailment, their first thought is probably, "I need to take a pill." For me, my first thought is, "What note will help mitigate this issue?" That is because I have had a lifetime of personal success stories using frequency to alter the form and function of my body.

Sound is completely non-invasive. You don't have to eat, swallow, or digest anything. There is no poking or prodding. All you have to do is listen and hum along.

Our bodies are frequency generators and receivers. Every cell in the body emits a frequency. Every cell in the body receives frequency. We are a symphony of sound and music that needs tuning from time to time. Every cell in the body also has an electrical charge – 72 millivolts is normal for healthy cells. Cells that have lower voltage are susceptible to disease.

You may be wondering how I became a believer in the power of sound as it relates to our physical and emotional health. I have some personal experiences to share with you from my own trial and error experiments with sound as a healing energy. I've been blessed to have been a part of four miracles in my life, so far. Three of them utilized the sound of my voice. The fourth was a very deep silent meditation.

I want to tell you the stories of these miraculous moments and the techniques that I used. I want you to see that when you know the ingredients of a miracle, you can create that magical miraculous space within which alignment is possible.

I stopped my professional career as an orchestral musician and teacher around the age of 40. I felt that I had a connection to music and sound that went beyond the symphony orchestra. I knew the power of music to lift people's spirits and change moods from playing hundreds of orchestral performances in front of appreciative audiences. Still, I felt that I had more to discover about sound and music than playing perfectly in tune, perfectly in rhythm, and perfectly in balance with the rest of the orchestra.

I took my fine-tuned listening abilities and turned them inward to rediscover the source of my sound. The journey brought me peace and a new sense of direction. Having moved through the ingredients of crafted "classical" melody, harmony, and structure, I found the power, beauty, and healing properties of tone and harmonics.

Unconsciously and intuitively, I knew that music would be my vehicle to self-realization. But somewhere in that left-brained labyrinth of discipline that paved the path to "classical" perfection, I lost the joy of the toy trumpet under the Christmas tree. I had lost the forest for the trees. What brought me back were questions. The nagging inner echo of the "why" brought me back. They pulled me back inside to find the patiently waiting though long forgotten **simple joy.**

I know now that this joy was never meant to be the unattainable reward in the never-ending pursuit of perfection! It was and is a GIFT! It's a byproduct of the creative process implanted in our souls to assure the eventual reconnection to our ultimate raison d'être.

In its purest sense, this gift of joy is of unspeakable worth. By opening to it for what it is, any and all Outer qualifiers fade into unreality. Once this connection is made within, even the simplest of sounds spring forth full of joy, purpose, empowerment, and healing. Healing first for ourselves and then for others.

A simple tone, made sacred with intention, is a powerful carrier wave for healing and enlightenment. It can have a harmonizing effect on our subtle life force energies. It can break emotional and psychological blocks and stimulate memory. It can carry us into deep meditative states of bliss where the barriers of time, space and mass do not exist.

Sound is one of the most basic components of the creative process. Recall that, "In the beginning, God **said**, 'Let there be light.'" It was the vibration that created light. As co-creators, as instruments of the ONE, we must sing whatever song comes most naturally to us. It is a fitting response to a Sacred Gift.

Sound is divine. Sound can alter the form and function of our bodily processes. I came to be a believer in the power of sound to change the form and function of the body by a leap of faith.

My first *Aha!* moment came when I turned 40 years old and was diagnosed with asthma. I hated the medicine and inhalers that made me feel so jittery. I decided to hum notes until I found one that really vibrated my lungs. After experimenting for a while, I found it. It happened to be A-flat/ G-sharp. I played the A-flat into the horn, and while I was sustaining that note, I sang an E-flat into the mouthpiece. This created a harmonic chord that really vibrated my lungs even more than just humming. I discovered that when I played this harmonic chord for 20 minutes a day that **I no longer had to use my inhalers. My asthma eventually went away**, I didn't have to play that chord anymore, and I was a believer in the power of sound for healing.

Remember that I am a person who likes to play with sound. Most people would take a pill, but I would rather listen to a sound than take a pill. This harmonic chord seemed to clear my lungs most naturally, like a cut healing, I didn't "feel" anything but better. To this day, many people who have had their ailments remediated by sound frequencies say, "It couldn't have been the sounds, I didn't feel anything!" I believe that is because the sound triggers our body's natural healing ability. And like a cut healing on your hand, you don't feel anything. It's the body setting itself right again because even though it lacked the biochemical energy to make the repairs in my lungs, it had the sound energy to use in its place.

Everything is frequency.

Frequency is at the essence of a thing, and the brain knows just how to use it.

I think the body/brain is always going through a kind of triage. The body/brain knows it has all of these tasks: making new cells, repairing old cells, digesting, eliminating, etc. If the body only got X amount of sleep and X amount of nutrition and was under X amount of stress, some tasks got put on the back burner. My body didn't have enough biochemical nutrients to make the repairs, so my brain recognized the sound energy frequencies and used them to make the repair instead.

The brain is a frequency modulator. It is like a radio tuner. It is constantly monitoring the frequencies in the environment and even the frequencies of the food that we eat. When we close our eyes and hold a banana in our hands, the brain knows by the banana's frequency that it's a banana. Yes, the brain hears the banana. It also smells it and sees it and feels it in the hand. The brain takes in information from all of the senses.

A person's intelligence could be measured by the amount of information a person takes in from all the senses simultaneously. The ability to assimilate as many senses as possible at once is a good definition of intelligence. Assimilate means to identify, process, and store information for retrieval at will later in time. The brain is constantly taking in information from our voice and ears and converting it to information which is carried by the nervous system to all parts of the body.

I also used the sound of my voice to tone my thyroid which had been underactive due to Hashimoto's. I did simple toning for five minutes a day with my voice, and it lowered the TSH levels from 17 to 6.58 in 2 weeks. I have the blood work to prove it. I understand that 6.58 is still a high level of TSH, but I had no adverse symptoms of a slow thyroid and it was a great improvement from 17!

Over the years, I have also totally repaired bulging discs in my lower back and neck using sound frequencies and avoided surgery. I have helped people who were scheduled for surgery for carpal tunnel, torn rotator cuffs, and torn meniscus to cancel their scheduled surgery. It was no longer needed because I was able to simulate the balancing frequencies for the out of balance sounds that came from their vocal prints with an audible tone for them to listen to which gave the body the energy it needed to fix the problem.

Sound has amazing positive effects on our bodies. It is completely noninvasive. It can trigger our body's natural healing abilities.

Sound gives power to things. Speaking a thought makes the thought tangible. The thought is no longer invisible and silent. Speaking it gives it substance, gives it a "body" and allows it to take up space and exist. That is the power of sound. Sound gives shape to matter. The number of cycles per second that a piece of matter vibrates determines its shape. A Google search of "making sound waves visible" will return with all kinds of equipment, both technical and man-ual, from tonoscopes to metal plates and tone generators. The science of seeing sound waves is called Cymatics. I created a simple tonoscope using an old hatbox from my grandmother. Instead of the hatbox top, I used some stretchy material across the top for the grains of salt to bounce around on. I cut a hole in the sidewall of the hatbox and inserted a piece of hose. When I sang into the hose, the salt made the sound waves visible as they changed shape with each pitch I blew into the hose.

Search "Cymatics" on YouTube, and you'll see plenty of examples of how sound creates the structure of matter.

Here is the process I used for Immune Support Har-monics and proof that sound affects matter. Every day, I did the same ten-minute morning meditation. I played long tones on my horn. This practice trained both my chops and my breathing. It was a win, win. While I was keeping my chops in shape, I was also playing and sustaining harmonic chords that sent me into meditation. Those chords boosted my immune system to the point that I could fight off colds and flu viruses with ease.

I recorded a harmonic audio file download to Boost the Immune Systems Response to Infections. The Immune Boosting audio file is available at www.thesoundlady.com. It only takes ten minutes a day to listen and hum along to this audio file from your computer or cell phone.

I published this case study years ago using an aura imaging camera to measure the changes in vibrational frequencies of the various organs and systems of my body as I played the harmonics on my horn. With each biological process – circulation, digestion, elimination, respiration – the software showed that after playing the harmonics, the energy of each system had accelerated and was vibrating at a higher frequency.

To see these photos in color go to my YouTube channel: https://www.youtube.com/watch?v=e76tbHcG5Xw

Horn and Voice Harmonics Effects on Aura
Before Playing Harmonics

Application of BioAcoustic theory for notes which govern specific biological processes as detected by an Aura Imaging Camera using Aura Imaging Software

The following pictures represent the changes in the aura while playing horn and voice harmonics to enhance specific biological processes.

Explanations of the state of each aura is provided by the Aura Imaging Software of Redwood City California.

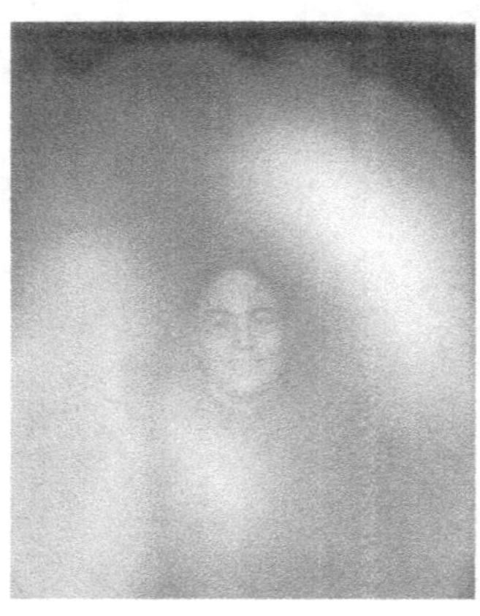

Horn and Voice Harmonics Effects on Aura
Before   Circulation-Heart

First we took a picture of my aura.

I played my horn and sang into it simultaneously creating harmonics corresponding to the processes of large and small circulation for @ 3 minutes and then took another aura picture.

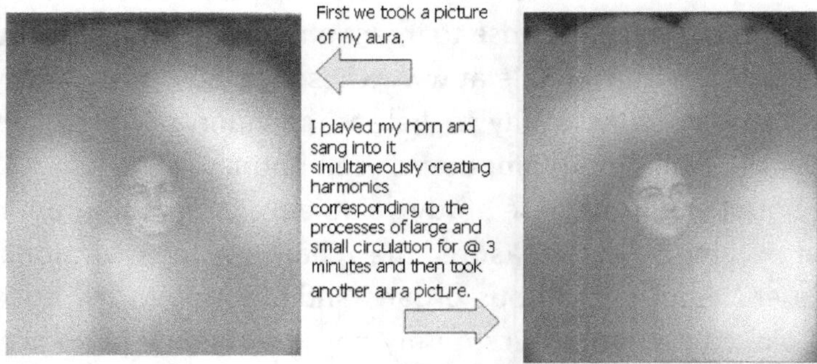

•The vibration of the Heart chakra accelerated from the frequency correlating to the color Blue to the frequency correlating to the color Violet. (Violet =glowing with magical spiritual inner light and guided by a higher power)

Horn and Voice Harmonics Effects on Aura
Before   Digestion-Solar Plexus

I played my horn and sang into it simultaneously creating harmonics corresponding to the processes of digestion for @ 3 minutes and then took another aura picture

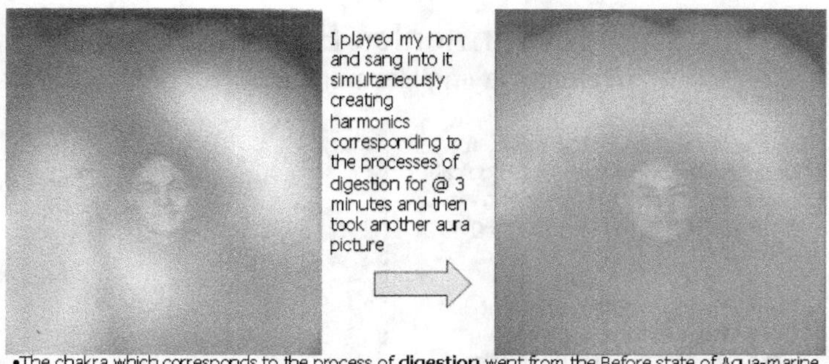

•The chakra which corresponds to the process of **digestion** went from the Before state of Aqua-marine (feeling a calm satisfaction)

• to Magical Blue   (Being in an intense state of beauty harmony and oneness with the divine. Spiraling out of my center is a beautiful healing energy creating myself as a clear conduit for healing myself and others.)

Horn and Voice Harmonics Effects on Aura

Before   Respiration-Throat and Heart

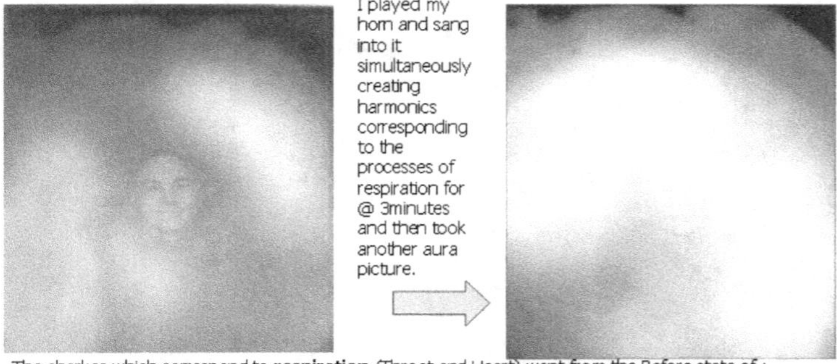

I played my horn and sang into it simultaneously creating harmonics corresponding to the processes of respiration for @ 3minutes and then took another aura picture.

The charkas which correspond to **respiration** (Throat and Heart) went from the Before state of :
Throat- Violet (radiating a magical inner peace) to Magical Violet (expressing the possibility of miracles)

Heart- from Blue (desiring peace and quiet) to Violet (glowing with magical spiritual inner light inspiring others and proving anything is possible.)

BEFORE PLAYING HEART HARMONICS | AFTER PLAYING HEART HARMONICS

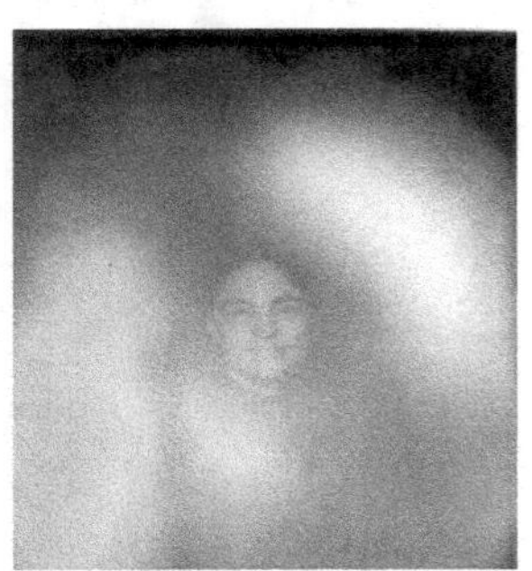

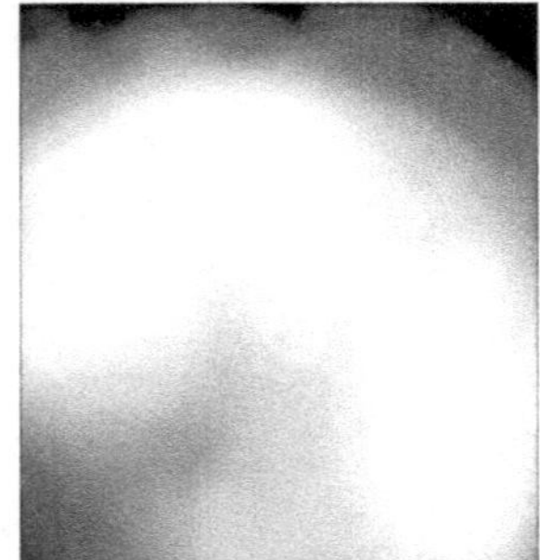

Chapter 4

Nitric Oxide

Paranasal Health

Now that we have seen that specific sounds can affect specific pieces of matter in the human body, let's talk for a minute about Nitric Oxide (NO). This is information from an article by the National Institute of Health. It's from a study done in 2002 about Nitric Oxide and our nasal passages. It is highly relevant to today's current coronavirus pandemic: [https://pubmed.ncbi.nlm.nih.gov/?term=high+nitric+oxide +production+in+human+paranasal+sinuses].

What is Nitric Oxide? It's nitrogen oxide which in humans is a signaling molecule in many physiological and pathological processes. It was proclaimed the "Molecule of the Year" in 1992. The 1998 Nobel Prize in Physiology or Medicine was awarded for discovering nitric oxide's role as a cardiovascular signaling molecule. **The most important information is that Nitric Oxide inhibits the replication cycle of severe acute respiratory syndrome coronavirus.** The study measured how simple humming increased Nitric Oxide in our nasal passages and sinuses. These are the tissues where coronaviruses linger for days before infecting other tissues.

Humming greatly increases nasal Nitric Oxide! It sounds too simple, but humming can kill coronavirus infections in our sinuses and nasal passages before it can wreak havoc on our lungs and throats. The American Journal of Respiratory and Critical Care Medicine published an article in 2002 with this exact finding about humming.

Another study from 1995 published in a natural medicine journal finds that "...**together with the well-known bacteriostatic effects of NO, [there is] a role for NO in the maintenance of sterility in the human paranasal sinuses...**"

Other studies on the paranasal sinuses as reservoirs for nitric oxide found that humming for one hour daily for four days stopped chronic rhinosinusitis.

How to Hum to Create More Nitric Oxide in Your Sinuses

Put your fingers on your sinuses under your eyes on both sides of your nose– little finger closest to your nose.

Start humming on a note in the middle of your vocal range.

Hum up in a scale-like manner or using a slow glide to find the note or notes that vibrate your sinuses the most.

Hum those notes for at least five minutes and you should feel your sinuses starting to drain.

Of course, you can always just hum your favorite song over and over or a children's song like "Mary had a Little Lamb" or "Row, Row, Row Your Boat"- pick a song that is easy for you to hum and hum it for 5 minutes. Chances are, some of the songs you will be humming will be a part of your vocal range that will vibrate your sinuses. It will create more Nitric

Oxide in your sinuses and stop the replication of CORONA-virus germs.

Immune Support Humming Technique

Using your voice, start on the middle C note (256Hz), slowly glide up with your voice sounding all the possible notes up to the C and an octave higher (512Hz) like you might on a penny whistle or a slide whistle.

Take a breath and then glide down from the high C (512hz) to the lower C (256Hz) Repeat these two steps for five minutes.

To find the sound of the note C, use onlinetonegenerator.com or a Chromatic C to C Pitch Pipe or any musical instrument you have handy.

While doing this, you are sounding all the notes of the sound spectrum of the C octave. These are the sounds I created with the French horn and my humming in the aura imaging camera case study that significantly raised the frequency of my body's systems and organs.

There are other ways to find the notes that vibrate the sinuses using your personal chakra scale notes, and we will go into more detail on this later.

Chapter 5

Toning

Consciously Using Natural, Unconscious, Body Sounds

Toning is using your voice to consciously express what your body is feeling. It is natural for the body to make sounds to release energy. It is how we are made. Our bodies make noises like burps, sighs, cries, and groans. When the body is releasing energy, it makes a sound. The sounds that come out of our mouths, whether words or groans, release our energy into the world.

We know how to groan, sigh, and cry instinctively without thinking about how. We didn't need to be taught these things. Unless we consciously stop the process, they just happen.

Have you ever had thoughts that you were afraid to say out loud? Maybe you knew they would not be accepted by your friends or that people would not like you if they heard you say certain things. Maybe we don't say certain things out loud because we don't want to believe that we have those thoughts. Maybe we can't bear to hear our true feelings.

There is something about **speaking a thought that makes it real**. Sound is the source of our creative power.

Creation stories throughout ancient traditions, including Christianity, identify sound as the primal creative force.

As far as toning is concerned, sound is where an abstract idea meets a manifested idea.

To quote Sharry Edwards, creator of the emerging science of Human BioAcoustics, "If you can moan, you can tone."

Moaning is a type of toning. The sounds we make when we moan calm the body. Humming is also a type of toning. If you think about it, we only hum for ourselves. It is a type of self-soothing. We might hum for an infant that we have in our arms, but that is one of the few instances where we use humming for someone else. Mostly humming is just for us!

There is great power in the sounds we make. A sound that is filled with intention and emotion can change us at the cellular level. Many emotions can get stuck in our bodies when we don't take the time to express and notice them. Let's say that a physical condition was fixed with sound or biochemical medicine or fixed with a change in diet and life-style. All symptoms left and the person was considered healed. But, if the physical condition was caused by an emotion that was trying to get attention in order to bring some-thing valuable to consciousness, then something will eventually re-trigger it and the symptoms will return.

Emotions can trigger symptoms. That's why it is impor-tant to use intention and emotional energy to clear the initial cause of the ailment from the emotional cellular memory. Using the consciousness of The Breath as a carrier wave for a heartfelt intention is a very useful sound healing tech-nique. Humming your personal chakra scale notes is another way to clear stuck, unconscious, emotional cellular memory.

Chapter 6

Humming

Giving Voice to a Sigh

Humming is something that we do for ourselves. We don't perform hums! Humming is a way of soothing ourselves, it's a kind of toning. There isn't as much stigma or judgment around humming as there is for singing. Many school children who have trouble hearing pitches are often told by their choral directors to just mouth the words instead of singing so as not to ruin the sound of the group. That experience, or others like it, generally discourages children from trying to sing a melody. Even to this day, it is hard to find a general music or chorus teacher who knows how to help children who can't match pitches with their voices.

Audiologist Dorinne Davis insists that everyone should be able to match musical pitches. If you can't, there is some kind of disconnect between the voice, ear, and brain. She has devised testing protocols for figuring out where the disconnect is and how to fix it. She is an internationally famous audiologist who taught me that the voice can't sound what the ear doesn't hear.

If you keep your mouth closed, like you do while humming, the sound vibrations stay inside your body. Our bones can conduct the sounds to all parts of the body. You'll know if you are full-spectrum humming when you feel the hum from your head to your butt. Opening the back of your throat like when you say the vowel "EEEE" can really get your ears ringing. Using different vowel sounds will project the hum up or down in your body. Vowel sounds like "Uhhh" or "Ohhh" open the back of the throat and send the sound down your spine. "Ahhh" is a very heart-centered sound. "AAAA," "IIII," and "EEEE" send the sound from the throat up towards your head.

Try a few hums and feel the effects in your body!

Tongue placement in the mouth while humming can amplify the power of the hum. You can hum with your teeth lightly touching by moving the sound of the hum to the front of the mouth and actually feel your teeth vibrate. As your teeth are connected to the meridians or energy pathways in the body, vibrating them sends energy down these pathways. Also, arching the tongue up and down in the mouth from back to front while humming a note creates harmonics inside your mouth which creates more frequency information for your brain to utilize.

Sharry Edwards teaches that the sounds coming from the voice are biofeedback information to the brain about the health of the body.

Humming is a wonderful way to provide the brain with useful frequencies to keep the body healthy. It's not something you do in public, so there is no one around to judge the quality of your humming. This judgment-free sound is soothing for your body. One of the reasons it is so good at calming you down is that humming creates more serotonin. Plenty of serotonin in your system keeps you very relaxed, whereas too much serotonin causes you to be more combative. It regulates the intensity of our emotional responses.

Humming is great for clearing your sinuses and making more Nitric Oxide, but it also has been proven to downward regulate blood pressure. Humming and sustained toning trigger the release of endorphins which are made by the Pituitary gland. They are responsible for a feeling of euphoria often associated with runner's high. The internal vibrations created while humming bring increased circulation and the tingly feeling of oxygenation.

I find it very effective when dealing with the head area of the body to try to engage the teeth while humming. As you hum, bring your lower jaw and teeth as close to the upper teeth as you can. As your teeth barely touch, you can feel them vibrating which sends the sound energy through all the meridians that are connected to our teeth.

If you search Google for Tooth Organ Chart you will find many of them. They usually show you the correlations between the teeth and organs, body parts, spinal segments, and glands. Here is a chart that shows glands, which will become useful when you know your chakra notes. Humming the chakra note that correlates to the gland you are working with makes the tooth/teeth vibrate and really enhances the energy to that gland. For example, if you were working with your Thyroid gland (Throat and 3rd Eye chakras), and you knew your personal chakra scale, you would hum those chakras note while barely touching your top and bottom teeth 3&30 and 14&19 for the thyroid hormones T3 and T4 and teeth 1&16 for anterior pituitary hormone TSH.

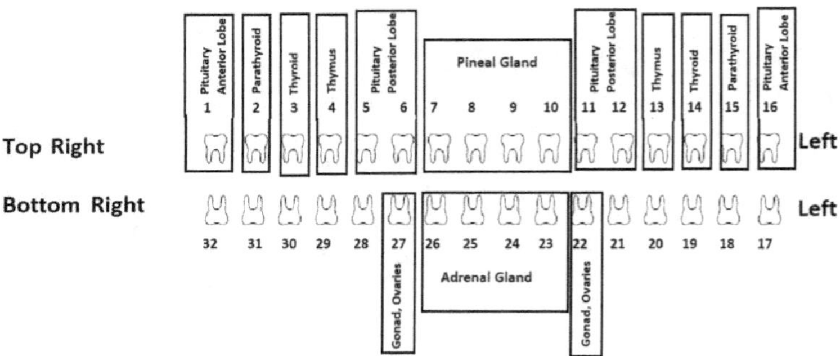

Chapter 7

Mantras

Word Toning

Mantras are a type of toning that can change repetitive thought patterns. This is sometimes also called chanting.

Repetition of a chant or mantra creates a groove, like those in a record, like a pathway of a thought-form in your mind. The more you repeat it, the deeper the groove, the stronger and surer the path. Chanting a mantra with an open heart will embed within your psyche an emotion that will be automatically triggered whenever the situation and need arises.

Mantras became a staple in my own life after having a life-altering experience using them. The story goes like this.

I found that I was obsessing about a person. I didn't like the feelings I had when I was obsessively thinking about this person. It was a situation that was impossible, and I could never have a relationship with this person for a myriad of reasons. Nonetheless, I was obsessing about being with this person. So, I created a mantra and made a little melody out of it. I recorded it and played it over and over for about two weeks. Then, I noticed that whenever I began to think about that person, the melody and lyrics I had written to counteract those thoughts started playing in my head. It was as if the mantra canceled out the old thought pattern and replaced it with the new one. It just disappeared.

That piece was called, **"Let It Go,"** and it's on my CD, **Prayer Songs**.

https://thesoundlady.com/product/prayer-songs-meditation-cd/

This modality can be used in many situations. For example, if you are angry because someone has caused you harm, and you meditate with this chant, after a while, whenever thoughts of anger toward that person arise, this chant will trigger in your memory. With it will come the feeling that you practiced and experienced while doing the chant. It's really good for breaking unwanted, no longer useful habits.

There are a couple of other mantra songs that are on the same CD called, **"The Forgiveness Chant,"** and, **"There Will Always be Enough."** It is always a good time for forgiveness. Holding onto old grudges does not help anyone. Forgiveness is something that we can learn and something that a lot of us need to learn as it does not always come naturally. Learning to forgive ourselves is often the first step in learning how to forgive others. This mantra song was very helpful in changing my mindset and heart set because it changed the pattern of my thinking.

The "Forgiveness Chant"

Forgiveness is a concept whose time has come. The underlying text to this melody is meant to be taken in the context of an oath:

With this sacred breath,
in the presence of all that is holy,

I do now,
in this eternal moment,
forgive,
forgive,
forgive
(myself, or fill in the blank with whatever or whoever you
want to forgive.)

This mantra is repeated three times in order to embed the melody in your mind for it to play over and over again. The way a mantra or chant works is that after you have repeated it over and over, whenever you begin to obsess over your forgiveness issue, the melody will begin to play in your head which helps you release your angry, unforgiving feelings.

"There Will Always Be Enough" Mantra

I wrote this when I was worried about money issues. It's a beautiful little melody with horn and piano that came to me in one clump. All of a sudden, the whole piece was in my mind. I quickly wrote it out on manuscript paper and recorded it. It very much helped me change my worrying approach to having what I needed. As with any mantra, repeat it three times over to embed it into your mind, and return to it often to lay the tracks of abundance.

Prosperity Mantra (sing this to the melody of the children's song BINGO)

All my needs are being met
Beyond my expectations.
Needs are being met,
Needs are being met,
Needs are being met
Beyond my expectations

Other Mantras

I'm still enough to listen, quiet enough to hear.
I'm still enough to listen, quiet enough to hear.
I'm still enough to listen, quiet enough to hear.
I'm still.

I'll always know.
What I need to know.
When I need to know it.

Make up your own Mantra

Use these simple concepts:

Rhythm

Decide if your mantra is needed to *disperse* energy or to *gather* energy.

Slow rhythms gather energy and faster rhythms disperse energy. Rhythms that are grouped in beats of threes (like a waltz) gather energy. Rhythms grouped in beats of twos (like a march) disperse energy.

Find or compose an affirming phrase that will re-pattern your thoughts.

Beat a drum or clap your hands to whichever rhythm you decide to use, fast or slow, and grouped in beats of two or three.

Say your affirming phrase over and over (the masters say to repeat it 5,000 times) while you beat out your rhythm.

Melody

If you know your root chakra note, sing the melody in that key. If you don't, I can help you find it!

Find or create a SIMPLE melody. Keep it simple so your brain doesn't have to think hard as you sing it. Sometimes you can use a melody from a familiar children's song, or you can make up your own melody in the rhythm of your phrase. Note that children's songs typically use the interval of a minor third because it is easy to sing. This interval also represents Yin and energy gathering and can easily be sung with beats grouped in either twos or threes, depending on how you space the lyrics.

Try "Ring Around the Rosy."

With a slow rhythm in groups of three beats: energy gathering.

RING A ROUND THE RO   SY
1 2   3, 1 2   3,   123, 123
POC KET FULL OF PO   SIE
12   3,   1 2   3   123, 123

With a fast rhythm in groups of two beats: energy dispersing:

RING A ROUND THE RO   SY
 1   2 1   2   12 12
POC KET FULL OF PO SIE
 1   2 1   2 12 12

Try "Mary Had a Little Lamb." This uses the interval of a major third which is more Yang, expansive, and dispersing. It has beats grouped in twos which are energy dispersing and can be sung at a fast tempo.

Ma ry had a lit tle lamb, lit tle lamb, lit tle lamb,
 1 2 1 2 1 2 1 2 1 2 1 2 1 2 1 2

Ma ry had a lit tle lamb who's fleece was white as snow
1 2 1   2 1 2 1   2   1   2   1   2 12

If there is a children's song whose melody matches the rhythm of your affirmative phrase, then use it. If not, compose your own simple melody. This will help you stay in a meditative mood where you are not overthinking.

Chapter 8

BioAcoustics

Sounds Made by Humans

For over 20 years now, I have been a BioAcoustic Practitioner. I have loved working with folks who have muscle injuries, mostly from overdoing it or from a sports injury. I found that BioAcoustics was a great protocol for painful muscles. Sharry Edwards created a frequency map of the human body that has the corresponding frequencies for all of the muscles. For each muscle, there is a specific frequency or frequency range, if it's a large muscle.

There are frequency combinations that can strengthen a weak muscle or relax a tight muscle. This comes in handy when the muscle can't be isolated because it is a part of a muscle group. If there is one muscle in a muscle group that is too tight, it is almost impossible to stretch only that muscle. Usually, if a muscle in a group is weak, other muscles in that same group are working overtime to support it. If some of them are too tight, then it is sometimes hard to get to the weak muscle. That's where the precision of BioAcoustics shines.

A frequency can be played that only affects that one weak muscle. The sound is non-invasive and doesn't require exercise!

I once did a BioAcoustic demonstration for a group of college sports doctors. A couple of hours before the meeting, I took the voiceprint of a student who had injured her hand and wrist during javelin practice. She had lost her footing and fell using her hand to brace her fall. Her right hand was much weaker than her left hand. Before I started playing her frequencies to strengthen the muscle of the hand that had been injured, I had her use a hand dynamometer. This is a device that when you squeeze it with your hand, it tells how much pressure you are using. First, we measured her left hand's strength and then the strength of her injured right hand and wrist. We noted the difference in strength between both hands and then I programmed a tone box that would generate the sounds specifically aimed at the muscles that were in stress according to her voiceprint.

She went off to class and got permission from her professor to listen to the sounds for an hour and a half during class. She then came to the meeting of sports doctors and fitness coaches with me. I explained my process to the doctors and showed them the results of the hand dynamometer comparison test. Now that the student had listened to the sounds for 90 minutes, we performed the dynamometer test again in front of the doctors. The second test showed that her injured right hand was now stronger than her left hand!

A healthy muscle is said to be *toned*. Muscle tone comes in three categories. Low muscle tone, normal muscle tone, and high muscle tone. Low muscle tone is like a rubber band that has been stretched out so much that it will no longer hold its original shape. It's saggy. Normal muscle tone allows the muscle to contract, expand, and return to its original shape. High muscle tone means muscles are really tight. Contracting and expanding this type of muscle is very painful.

Toned muscles allow you to have great posture. Your muscles can hold their shape in a passive position. When muscles are too weak or have low muscle tone, your muscles can't hold your body upright and erect. You tend to slouch. Muscle tone is essential for many normal body functions such as holding the spine erect, keeping the eyes open, keeping the jaw closed, and controlling incontinence, to name a few. One of my clients, an 83-year-old woman with incontinence, complained that she had to change her diaper twice a night. After one month of listening to her BioAcoustic sounds to strengthen the muscles of the pelvic floor, she was able to sleep through the night!

BioAcoustics is the emerging science that studies the sounds made by animals, birds, dolphins, and whales. Sharry Edwards has pioneered Human BioAcoustics for the last 30 years. Human BioAcoustics measures the frequencies in the human voice as a biofeedback system for the health of the body. We all have heard the sound of someone's voice change when they are tired, sick, or stressed. We have heard a teen-age male's voice change as he is going through puberty due to the hormones that are secreted to mature the male body. Our voices are perfect feedback systems for the brain.

There is an important connection between the voice, the ear, and the brain. The frequencies spoken by the vocal cords are sent through the cranial nerves which intertwine with the vocal cords and go right up to the brain. The vagus nerve travels up the body from the abdomen through the vocal cords and into the brain as the 10th cranial nerve. This nerve informs the vocal cords, and that information goes straight up to the brain. The sound of the voice is one of the ways that the brain knows the health of the body!

The state of our health is truly in the sound of our voice.

Human BioAcoustics records the sounds of a speaking

voice into a computer. The microphone intercepts the voice, and the computer tallies the exact same frequency information that the ears are hearing and sending to the brain.

Here we can see on a graph the energy of our body in terms of sound frequencies at the moment we are speaking. It's like taking a Polaroid snapshot of our energy at that moment. In the computer output, we can see the normal energy range for our voice. On the graph, normal vocal energy is in the dark gray section. Then, we can then identify the low energy frequencies and the high energy frequencies as compared to the normal range frequencies. From this information, we can see which frequencies the body does not have enough energy for and which frequencies the body is putting a lot of energy into as compared to the normal energy range of your voice.

BioAcoustics identifies the stressed frequencies in the voice – those with high or low energy compared to the rest of your voiceprint.

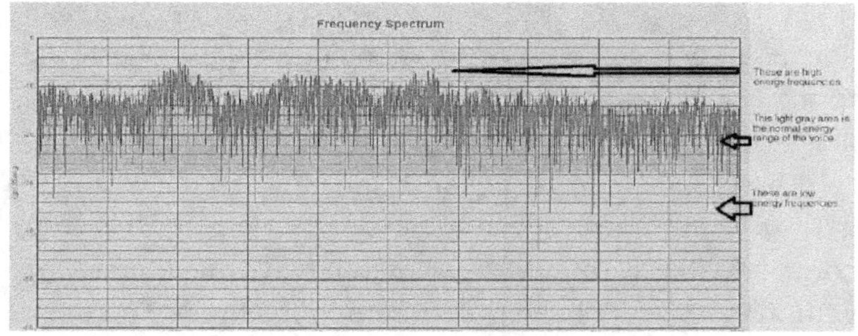

With a BioAcoustic database of thousands of voiceprints, Sharry Edwards put together a frequency map of the human body. With it comes the possibility to correlate the low or high energy frequencies with different body parts and chemicals: muscles, vertebrae, amino acids, enzymes, vitamins, cell salts, genes and their activators, proteins, pathogens, and toxins. When the analysis is complete, it is possible to identify what parts or systems of the body are lacking in energy. It's possible to see what parts or systems of the body are using the more energy. We can then balance those stressed frequencies by playing balancing sounds back to you through a low-frequency tone generator. Your brain hears the sounds and uses that pure sound energy to make the needed adjustments.

Yes, even if you have not had the right amount of nourishment or the right amount of sleep, or if you have been under a lot of stress, the brain will use the frequency to make the repair. The essence of everything is frequency. The language of the brain is frequency.

If the brain detects frequency information that is between 15 Hz and 20,000 Hz, the brain knows it is sound energy. If the brain detects frequencies from 400–790 THz (trillion Hz), it knows it is visual input. The brain doesn't actually need the physical/biochemical matter to be ingested into the body for it to work. If the hand is holding a banana, if the nose is smelling a banana, or if the eyes are seeing a banana, the brain knows there is a banana. If you played the tonal frequency of the banana, the brain would easily recognize it and prepare to use that sound energy information. This happens because the brain works with the frequency essence of matter as well as with the matter itself.

The sounds that we use to re-entrain the brain to a normal energy level are low-frequency sounds. They sound more like your refrigerator motor than music. They are frequencies at the bottom of the human hearing range. Bio-Acoustic Practitioners (BARA's – BioAcoustic Research Associates) use the Beta Brain Wave frequencies because that is the octave of brain waves where the brain is in its most active and alert mode. The sounds are usually between 16 and 32 Hz. The equipment that is used is very accurate. The high-quality vocal microphone that we use to record the voice needs to record to 0.03 Hz accuracy in that low range.

In other words, if the microphone recorded a stressed frequency with low energy at 427.54 Hz, a practitioner would need to balance that energy by playing it back to you. If the microphone was not accurate to the degree we require and the low frequency was really 428 Hz, playing back to you 427.54 Hz will not fix anything. If 428 Hz is the problem, we need to play 427.97 Hz to 428.03 Hz for your brain to use it for that specific issue.

The sounds that we play to balance the stressed frequencies are like little laser beams to the brain. The playback equipment has to be very accurate. We use a device that Sharry developed called a tone box. It plays analog frequencies accurately down in that very low range. We use analog frequencies because we have found that the brain much more readily uses analog sound to adjust the form and function of the body than digital sound.

According to Sharry's frequency equivalent database, if the frequency for calcium was accurately recorded as a low energy frequency at X Hz, then the tone box would have to be accurate to within 0.03 Hz to raise the energy level of calcium. Instead, if it played to X + 0.05 Hz or X − 10 Hz, then it would not do anything to the energy level of calcium.

Sharry Edwards is the Pythagoras of this millennia. In my opinion, her software and playback equipment along with her database of frequency equivalents is worthy of a Nobel prize for medicine.

Testimonials

These come from my past clients. As you can see, BioAcoustic voice analysis with low-frequency biofeedback is very effective for pain.

Chronic Neck Pain

"Kathleen, I have been bragging about you to anyone who will listen! My sound therapy with you has been a game-changer! My chronic neck, ear, and head pain that I have had for 15 years (since my car accident) is gone! Your next task is to help [a friend] with his chronic pain. We will be calling you when we return home to Santa Fe for you to set up sessions to help him. You are an Angel!"

Chronic Hamstring Pain

"I had a nagging pain in my left hamstring for two years and no matter how long I stretched it, it would not go away. At the end of the day, after teaching fitness classes, it was really a problem. I had to cut back on the running that I love because it just hurt too much. I had Kathleen analyze my voice recording and she found that the Gluteus Medius muscle was at the crux of the problem. Now, as a fitness trainer, I am trained to evaluate people by looking at their posture, etc., but you can't see the Gluteus Medius muscle. Her software found it to be an overly strong frequency and she programmed a sound into my tone box to help relax it. I also found some exercises to stretch that particular muscle and did them while I listened to the sounds. What a difference! The nagging pain went away after about a week and I have been pain-free ever since. Thanks, Kathleen!"

Arthritis Pain

"As a practicing nurse practitioner for over 35 years, I have been introduced to multiple treatment modalities for countless maladies. I am open to Western, Eastern—you name the origin—approaches to healthcare and promotion. I apply the scientific method to assess these options and their potential

healing or diagnostic potential. I have suffered the pain and disfigurement of advancing osteoarthritis of my hands and feet for nearly 20 years. Having lived with NSAIDs, cortisone injections, and pain while continuing to care for patients and enjoy the activities that bring joy to my life, one can only imagine my hopeful excitement when Kathleen introduced me to Sound Therapy…Within two days of listening to the tones she gave me, the pain in my hands and feet simply stopped. I was able to walk 18 holes of golf and have the energy for more. My fingers stopped aching and I was able to work in my glass studio, type on the computer, and work in the garden without paying the pain price I was so accustomed to. That was three full months ago, and I am still pain-free 95% of the time. Now, Kathleen is focusing on WHY the arthritis has attacked my joints, and, using the technology of sound, she has discovered a chemical imbalance in my ability to clear calcium from my body and to prevent it from accumulating in my joints…I see Sound Therapy as an exciting pathway to diagnosing and treating many issues. I see it as the true 'Wave of the Future' – one wave I intend to ride."

Torn Lateral Meniscus

"Surgeons said I would require surgery to heal the tear in my knee, but they were reluctant to operate due to my cancer diagnosis and resulting complications. After four weeks of listening to my sounds for 2-3 hours a day – which was easy to do because I was bedridden anyway – I was pain-free, weight-bearing, and had regained 100% of my range of motion. I no longer needed possibly risky surgery. I am very grateful for the opportunity to use BioAcoustics. It has not only helped with my knee but many other health issues over the past seven years. I would definitely recommend this blessing of a therapy to everyone!"

Chapter 9

Frequency = Energy

Dr. John Beaulieu, a sound healer who uses tuning forks in his practice, says, "Scientifically, an energy field is defined as a medium that connects two or more points in space, through energy expressed as tone or vibration."

Tone and vibration create an energy field. A high-frequency energy field, such as the type that is created by sacred sound, can create a state of perfection, harmony, and cooperation. Physics tells us energy never dies; it can be changed but it can't be killed. It is also a common acknowledgment in Quantum Physics that **Energy=Frequency**.

Frequency and vibration are the essence of energy. People say, "Everything is energy." Albert Einstein's famous equation proves this premise:

$$e = mc^2$$

Here, **e** is energy, **m** is mass, and **c** is the speed of light.

According to The Vitamin Lawyer, Ralph Fucetola, in his paper on vibration and frequency as nutrition, it would be more accurate to say, "Everything is frequency." Ralph explains that the formula can more precisely be rewritten as:

hn = mc2

He explains that the formula of energy is a wave. Energy (**e**) = **hn, h** being Plank's constant of action, and **v** being frequency. Planks' Constant is a unit of measurement in Quantum Physics. It links the amount of energy a photon carries with the frequency of its electromagnetic wave.

So, the energy of a wave is its frequency times this constant. It means we can substitute **hn** for their equivalent, **e**. Therefore, **hn = mc2.**

Since **h** and **c** are constants of Nature, and only **n** and **m** change, for every m there is an equivalent **n.**

For every mass, there is an equal frequency.

An energy field is a frequency field. The field can be changed, adjusted, and transformed by changing the frequency of the field. Resetting this field back to its perfection of harmony, cooperation, and balance can be accomplished by changing the frequency of the field. This causes a shift in the field, and that shift in the field can be responsible for miracles. Miracles are simply a phenomenon of physics that we do not yet completely understand.

A person with multiple personality disorder can have personalities that have a disease and other personalities that do not have that disease. One day they could have cancer, and the next day it's gone. Dr. Beaulieu says, "From an energy perspective, remission can take place instantly based on a field shift. When the new field emerges, endogenous biochemical cascades that destroy cancer cells appear naturally as part of the new field."

A very dear friend of mine had multiple personality disorder from a terribly abusive childhood. Children who are abused have seven times the normal rate of developing cancer. My friend got cancer in her 40's. The energetic fields of the personalities were drastically different. Some of the personalities had cancer, and some of them didn't. The ones who had cancer and wanted to die were always trying to sabotage the others who had cancer but wanted to live. They would "take over" the personality and do things like forget to take medication. I found it amazing that these personalities could switch back and forth with and without cancer instantly.

Energy can change, but it can't be destroyed or deleted. And it can change at an amazing speed as if someone flipped a switch when the need and opportunity presented itself.

Chapter 10

Three Ingredients of a Miracle
Four Miraculous Stories

I was part of a miraculous healing where the energy field shifted due to the drumming, singing, and chanting space that a group had created. The chant was about ONENESS. I learned it while meditating on the beach at the ocean in Orleans on Cape Cod. The person was cured of restless leg syndrome.

Before we get into that specific little miracle, I'd like to share my personal observations concerning miracles in general. Know that I have not studied any of the Miracle courses or read any books on miracles. This is just from my personal experience. After I had experienced or witnessed several miracle cures, I tried to find a common thread and I found there were three ingredients that seemed to exist at the time of the miracle:

1. An Open Heart
2. High Vibrational Emotional Frequency
3. The Awareness of ONENESS – Your Divinity

First, preparing for a miraculous state of mind requires an open heart. You can think about something that makes your heart smile. A puppy, an infant, a beautiful sunset. Whatever it is, focus on it and feel your heart opening. A broken heart is also an open heart. A broken heart is vulnerable and has been torn open by a loss of a loved one, for example. It feels like there is a hole in the heart where the old cords of connection once held fast. Now, they have been ripped away, and we indeed have an etheric hole in our hearts. This state of being can also be an opportunity for a miracle.

Second, with that open-hearted perspective, raise your emotional vibration and the frequency of the space you are in. For this particular miracle, I used drumming and chanting. You can also use dancing and hand clapping or body drumming with your hands. The louder and more resonant the sounds and an increasing rhythm will gradually raise your frequency and the frequency of the space you are in.

Third, merge into awareness of ONENESS. Connect with the ONENESS that permeates the consciousness of all that is. In truth, we are all connected in this web of ONENESS. In this Oneness state, we connect with our Divinity. Now, there are many ways to connect with our divinity. That is the special sauce. Opening the heart and raising your frequency are just a few of the ways you prepare for that Oneness state of mind and heart.

When I was in high school, my Religion teacher, who happened to be a Jesuit priest, gave us an unusually difficult homework assignment. He asked us to define God. To my 13-year-old mind, this was going to be fun. That night as I lie in bed pondering this ontological question of the ages, I finally came to a conclusion that I could live with. I thought, if you put all the love in the world together, that would be God. If we took all of the love that was in all of our hearts and all of the love that is evident in nature and put it together, that would be God.

Back in 1965, Quantum Physics was not yet a part of the world view, but Quantum Physics tells us that we are all connected in a web of etheric energy. When we try to access the consciousness of that etheric web, we find it is permeated with love in all the empty space. At least, that's what I found, and it gave credence to my young impression of God being all the love in everyone and everything.

To enter this Oneness mindset, we must forget about yesterday, forget about tomorrow, and forget about now. By just *being* in this space where we no longer identify with our individual egos, this space of oneness and connection allows us to enter our own sense of Divinity. Here, anything is possible.

Miracle Story #1 – Restless Legs No More

It was around the turn of the 21st century when I found myself caring for my wife who had breast cancer. She was disabled and not able to work. I was caring for her, working full time, walking the dog, running the house, and maintaining the yard. It was a very stressful time. One way I would relieve stress was to go to the ocean. My personal coping mechanism at the time was to go as long as I could until I felt I was about to break, then take a weekend at the ocean to release all the stress so I could go back and continue doing what needed to be done.

My wife, Marlo, had friends who had a condo near the beach in Orleans on Cape Cod. They had offered it to us for the weekend, just in time. I felt like I really needed to have a good cry, and I always liked doing that at the ocean. To me, the roar of the ocean was such an immense sound, and the ocean was so incredibly large that my little cries would not upset anything there. The ocean beach was a place for me that could absorb my feelings and not be any worse for the wear. I was always conscious about having strong feelings in places that would affect other people. I didn't like it when others spewed their angry venom near me, so I was always conscious about not doing that to others.

We got to the condo on a Friday night, had a great seafood meal, watched some TV, and then I went to bed. I was looking forward to going to the ocean in the morning for one of my ocean meditations and releases. I was disappointed when Marlo decided to stay up longer and not come to bed with me. She ended up falling asleep on the couch which is where I found her in the morning on my way out to the ocean. She was a late sleeper and not a morning person. I knew I would have several hours all to myself on the beach before she awoke.

I drove the short distance to the beach, parked the car, and walked out onto the sand. It was early morning, and there was no one else in sight. I found a place to situate myself in the soft, warm sand for a sitting meditation. My plan was to open my heart and let out the tears. I sat there for a while and to my surprise, no tears came. I was thinking about how upset I was that Marlo had not come to bed with me last night. Her being sick was slowly diminishing our relationship as she herself was shrinking inch by inch from this world. But still, no tears came.

I decided to stand up and start to do a walking meditation with my bare feet in the sand. I learned this type of walking meditation at the San Francisco Zen Center in a workshop by Pema Chödrön, an American Tibetan Buddhist. The Buddhists call it, "The Zombie Meditation Walk." As I walked, I focused on my feet and how they touched the sand and how the energy of the crystals in the sand was sending energy into my feet. I felt my energy going into the sand as I was very connected to the Earth.

Then, after about 30 minutes of doing this, I heard a verse in my head out of the clear blue:

I am the sand
I am the sun
I am the water
We are one

I was astonished and full of awe to hear this. I started repeating it over and over as I continued my walking meditation. Due to my propensity for playing with sound, I started to develop a melody around the words. After about another 30 minutes, I felt it was time to go back to the condo and share this experience with Marlo.

I arrived back at the condo, parked the car, and started walking to the porch. There was Marlo with a cup of coffee and a cigarette sitting on the front steps.

As I approached her, she smiled and rolled her eyes at me.

"What?" I said. "What are you laughing at?"

One of Marlo's many gifts was that she could see spirits and auras. "You've brought a whole parade of spirits with you back from the beach!" she said. "They're following you like the Pied Piper, all in a line behind you."

"Great!" I smiled. "Let's go make some music together with them."

I told her about the song and verse I was given on the beach while meditating and wanted to show her musically so she could hear it, too. She was game. We both went into the condo to get a drum, and on the way, I asked her why she had not come to bed last night. She said she was having one of her bouts with restless legs and didn't want to wake me.

I felt bad. She was actually being considerate by not coming to bed, and I had taken it that she would just rather watch TV. I shook my head at myself realizing that I had assumed something and got upset about it when it wasn't true.

We sat down with our drums and started improvising with the words and rhythms and melodies for this verse. We engulfed ourselves in this concept of ONENESS that the verse related with singing and drumming for about 20 minutes. Then she stopped.

"I'm having an incredible experience," she told me. "I just heard in my head that I will no longer have restless legs syndrome." As she heard this, she saw energy coming out of her legs and falling onto the floor.

"What does it look like?" I asked.

"Like gasoline in a puddle at a gas station," she told me. "Like that dirty, electric blue and murky yellow color."

We sat there for a while to let this sink in. My guess was that the spirits at the beach had taken a liking to me and wanted me not to be sad. They used the space that we created with the drumming and chanting of the ONENESS verse to cure Marlo of her restless legs – just like that! Cured!

She never again had restless legs, which, needless to say, perplexed her doctors.

Prior to this, Marlo had tried several medications to help with the restless legs as it was sometimes very stressful for her. Her whole body would jerk, her arms and legs would flail around every 30 seconds or so, and it would last for hours until she finally fell asleep exhausted. It was a miracle that she never experienced it again. It wasn't until after I had the experience of being involved in several other miracles that I understood the three common ingredients to create a space within which miracles were possible.

Miracle Story #2 – Dance of a Lifetime

A few months after Marlo died from a long, 10-year battle with breast cancer, I moved to Santa Fe, New Mexico. I drove across the country with my friend, Jim, the mystic. On the way through Oklahoma, we picked up his friend, Oro, another mystical, magical being. That was quite a fun ride!

I was about to start my new job as an Activities Director for a retirement community that was built to accommodate elder LGBTQ folks. It was founded by a very forward-thinking force of nature, Joy, who was also an ex-partner of my wife. Joy and Marlo had stayed friends all the years after their relationship had ended.

The retirement complex had apartments for average folks too, so it was quite a mix of interesting people. Some of them lived in their apartments or condos, but there were also many units made up of different levels of assisted living. I had an apartment to live in and a beautiful building to work in and was very happy there, while it lasted. There was a hostile takeover of the organization, bankruptcy soon followed, and my life got very interesting in Santa Fe. I was a house sitter, couch surfer, dog and cat sitter, acupuncture office manager, chiropractic office worker, and finally an Uber driver! That was just how Santa Fe worked – many people had two or three different jobs because there was really no industry in the city except for hospitality and art.

Also, I learned after being there a while, Santa Fe was a place that drew wounded healers to help us find our way and teach us how to ask for help. So many healers are on their own in communities where they have to hide their gifts. In Santa Fe, there are healers of all kinds. There are psychics, card readers, palm and foot readers, Shamans, astrologists, chiropractors, acupuncturists, naturopaths, osteopaths, and many multidimensional men and women, old and young, from all over the world. Jim, Oro, and I had landed in a place where we could ask many people to help us with our wounds and find a modality that was comfortable for us to work within. It was the perfect place for me at that time in my life. I was healing from the loss of the love of my life and ten years of caretaking that had left me depleted. I knew that if

I was half as good at taking care of myself as I was at taking care of Marlo that I would be fine.

A couple of months into the job, I decided to attend the Friday night cabaret at the nightclub inside the main building of the retirement community. There was a very talented gay man playing the piano and singing on stage. Charles had his own unique style. He was a classically trained pianist, and let me tell you, he tickled every key on that piano! He played waltzes and jazz standards, and wow, he could sing! What a voice! Performing for this crowd, he was in his glory. People were dancing and very much enjoying the safe place to congregate and let their hair down.

I wasn't having as good a time as everyone else. I was missing Marlo and remembering how she could dance the shoes off of anyone I had ever met. I missed dancing with her. Feeling sorry for myself amidst all of this reverie, I decided to go back to my apartment and call it a night. As I walked back to my apartment, my back started to ache. I had a long history of low back pain, but I couldn't think of any reason why my back should be hurting. I hadn't done anything that would have strained it. I hadn't even danced!

As I climbed the stairs, the pain got more and more intense. I barely made it to my bed and tried to find a comfortable position. Since I had not done anything to cause the low back pain as far as I could figure out, I realized there must have been an emotional trigger. I went into meditation to see if I could get to the bottom of it and heal it, once and for all. I began to look back on all the situations in my past where I found myself disabled and out of work due to back pain. I thought if I could find the common denominator to all of these situations, I would be onto something.

I pondered and meditated and finally came to the awareness that the feeling of isolation was the common denominator to all of the past experiences I had with debilitating back pain. It seemed that whenever my back would "go out," I was feeling very alone and isolated. I went deeper into meditation and it became obvious that my feelings of isolation were just an illusion. I was able to embrace the knowing that I was never alone. I spent a long time meditating on the oneness of all things and the feeling of isolation left my heavy heart. I was at peace and fell asleep with the awareness of a very slight tingling in my lower back. That slight tingling was there most of the night. It went from my lower back down my legs and into my feet. It wasn't enough to keep me awake, it was just a minimal, barely noticeable feeling of tingling.

When I woke up the next morning, I felt very refreshed. I rolled out of bed, put both feet on the floor, and noticed something very different. Both legs were exactly the same length, and I could put complete weight on them both with no pain. This was very new. Inflammation in the past had caused my hips to torque making one leg longer than the other by an inch or so, which was enough to cause a lot of pain when I walked, sat, and stood. I felt that Marlo had been helping from the ethers to heal my lower back all night long, and I was amazed by my newfound flexibility. This was a miracle for me. I have never had low back pain again since that night, and although this would be a good place to end this story, it gets even better.

Two weeks later, I decided to go again to the Friday night cabaret. I vowed to myself that I would dance, that I would ask someone to dance and I was going to have a great time just like everyone else.

The night was wearing on and I was at a table of new friends. A couple of us went to the bar to refresh our drinks where we started up a conversation with another woman at the bar who seemed to be there with a man who wasn't paying much attention to her. This woman asked my friend to dance. My friend declined as she was there with her girl-friend and wasn't in a dancing mood. I saw that this was my chance, so I asked her if she would dance with me instead. She agreed. We went to the dance floor as the pianist started playing a song that I knew. I can't remember now what it was, probably just a karaoke standard, but I remember that I knew it well. That always makes dancing easier, when you know the rhythms, the melody, and the lyrics to the song. We were the only ones on the floor at the time, and all eyes were on us. This didn't bother me, but my dancing partner had a little bit too much to drink and was a little wobbly. I did something then that was very uncharacteristic for me; I put my arm around her waist, and I pulled her close to me so we could dance and she wouldn't fall.

That was bold, Kath, I thought to myself. *Where did that come from?*

I felt like I was dancing on air. I was doing things on the dance floor that I had never done before. I was just moving to the rhythms and phrases, improvising as I went, grace-fully leading my dance partner around the floor. Every move just morphed into the next, always in perfect sync with the phrasing of the song. My partner and I were like one unit, perfectly in sync. Our audience was entranced by our sym-metry. During his piano interlude, even Charles saw us danc-ing and mentioned how beautiful the dancing was while he was playing. When the song was over, everyone applauded, and several of the older gay men asked me to please dance with them. I said yes to one of them and started dancing with him, but he was clearly too old and fragile to be danc-ing. He almost lost his balance and fell, but a couple of his friends were hovering nearby to catch him.

I went back to the table where I was sitting, and everyone was abuzz about my dancing! One friend mentioned to me that she had not seen that side of me before. I was the center of attention, performing for all to see. My friend's experience of me up to that point in time was that I was someone who preferred to be in the background as an observer and listener. I admitted that it was a bit uncharacteristic of me to do what I had just done.

Soon after, I left the cabaret and walked back to my apartment to fall into a blissful sleep. When I awoke the next morning, I felt like I had been hit by a mac truck! It was funny, that was an expression that Marlo used to explain to me how she felt after getting her chemo infusion. I rarely used it, but it came to me then, and I finally put two and two together.

Last night, Marlo's spirit had entered my body on the dance floor, and she danced me. She *danced* in me, she danced as me, she was dancing with me and leading like she always did. I knew this to be true. I was also exhausted having toasted all my circuits the night before, raising to the frequency that allowed her to become one with me. The entire day, all I could do was look forward to going back to sleep. Looking back on it now, what an extraordinary experience that was! My back was healed, and I got to dance with my wife for one last time. Life was good!

Miracle Story #3 – Activating the Earth's Crystal Grid

I had been in Santa Fe for a couple of months and was really feeling at home in the energy of such a magical place. I was meditating daily, and in one of my meditations, I had a "knowing" or what I call it when all of a sudden, I know something that there is no logical reason for me to know. It wasn't that I heard a voice say anything, it was just a kind of feeling that felt important. It felt like something I should pay attention to, so I did.

What my inner prodding was suggesting was I needed to find a new- age bookstore. I felt there was a book in a bookstore that I was meant to read. Which one? I didn't know. I started by asking friends to point me to a local new age bookstore. They all said the same thing, "You should go to The Ark bookstore."

On my next day off from work, I drove on over. I thought, *Okay, now that I'm here, which book am I supposed to read?* I moseyed around and got a feeling for all of the isles, and after about an hour, I settled on a new book by Gregg Braden, who lived in Santa Fe, *Deep Truth – Igniting the Memory of Our Origin, History, Destiny, and Fate*. I went back home and started reading. As I got through the first couple of chapters, I started to feel that the book was really not speaking to me in the way I thought it would. I was ready to rethink my process, and then there it was.

He was talking about a trip he had taken to Chaco Canyon in the four corners area where New Mexico, Colorado, Utah, and Arizona meet. He said that just walking on that land he could, "feel the crunch of the crystal sand beneath his feet." After I read that, I knew I was supposed to do something at Chaco Canyon, and the second part of the adventure began.

I went back to the bookstore and started searching for the next book that would tell me what I was supposed to *do* in Chaco Canyon. After browsing for a while, I found a new book by Dolores Cannon, *The Three Waves of Volunteers and The New Earth*. What a read! It was on page 427 where I found what I was looking for. There was a short chapter in the book that Dolores said she felt compelled to insert into the book even though few people would be interested in it. She knew there was a small group of people on the planet who needed to see this information. The chapter was called, *The Keepers of the Grid*.

After reading it, I *knew* I was one of the Grid Keepers and that I had a job to do ASAP. I knew I was to go to Chaco Canyon and reactivate the portion of the Earth's crystal grid that had been damaged eons ago when Atlantis was destroyed. Today, the crystal grid network that ran all around the planet was in grave need of repair as we were once again experimenting with "dark matter" using the Collider experiments, and we were putting the Earth in danger again. With the crystal grid network restored around the planet, the Earth would be able to activate her 3rd strand of DNA which would take her and all of us into the new, evolving 5th-dimensional consciousness that is our destiny. I was supposed to go to Chaco Canyon (about a three-hour drive) and reactivate the broken part of the crystal grid there.

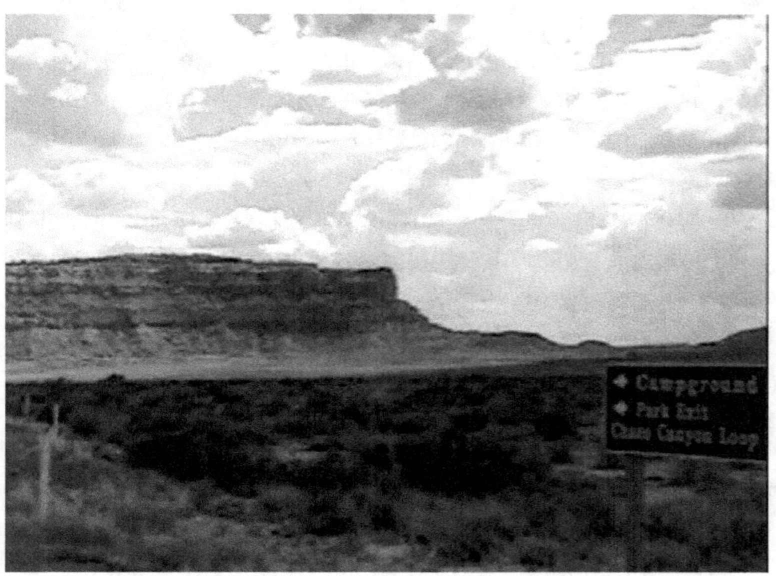

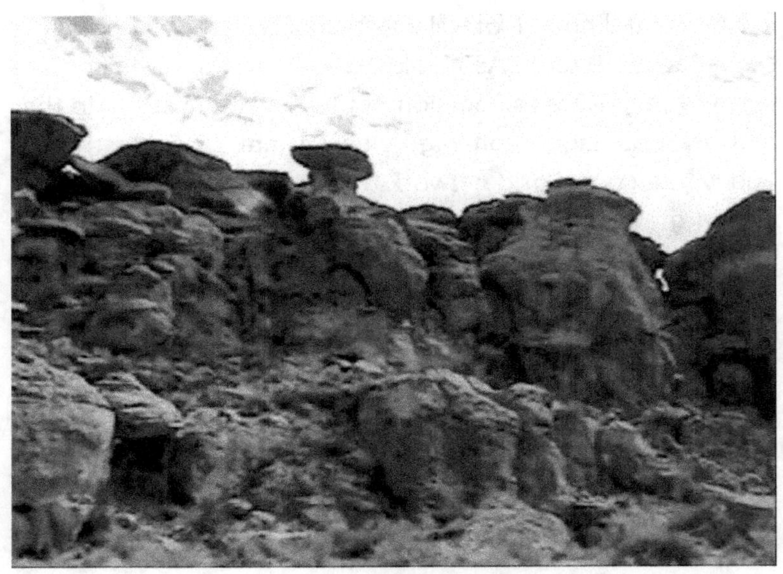

On my next weekend off, I planned the long day trip. I knew it would take three hours to get there and three hours to get back, but I didn't know how long it would take me to fix the crystal grid or where to find it. It was going to be a long day. I brought snacks, my horn, my seven-chakra drum, a pendulum, a video camera, and lots of water. After a long ride, I finally arrived at the end of a 12-mile long dirt road that led into the canyon, I couldn't believe the vastness of the place.

The directions I received from the book said these crystals that I needed to repair were usually near water. There was no water anywhere to be seen. It was desert-like. An ancient culture once thrived here, but that was long ago. The land had been abandoned for many years.

I sat and meditated for a while. During my meditation, I felt that the people of this ancient city were not gone at all. They were still there, in a parallel dimension. I could hear children and people talking. I was at the water's edge. Men were fishing. I could see that this was once a thriving community around a large mass of water.

Satisfied with the etheric water that I was experiencing, it was all proof enough for me. I was confident that I was in the right place to do this work though I didn't know where to start. I picked up a map of the ancient settlement and sat down at a picnic table with my peanut butter and jelly sandwich and my pendulum. I held the pendulum over the map.

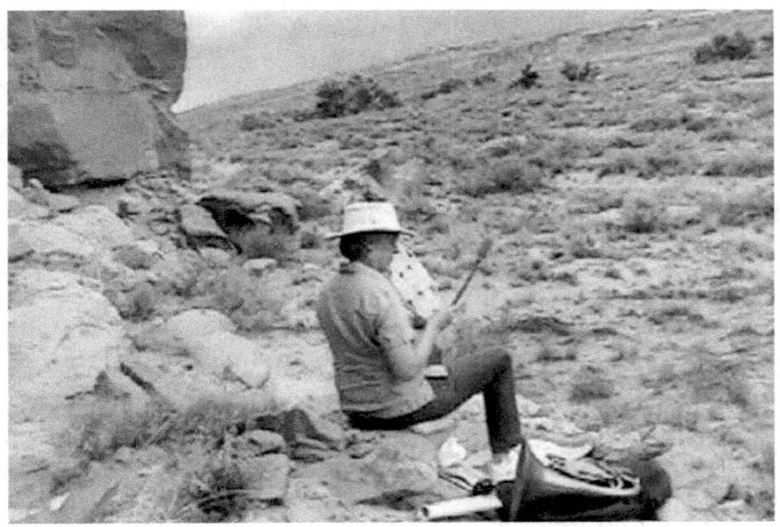

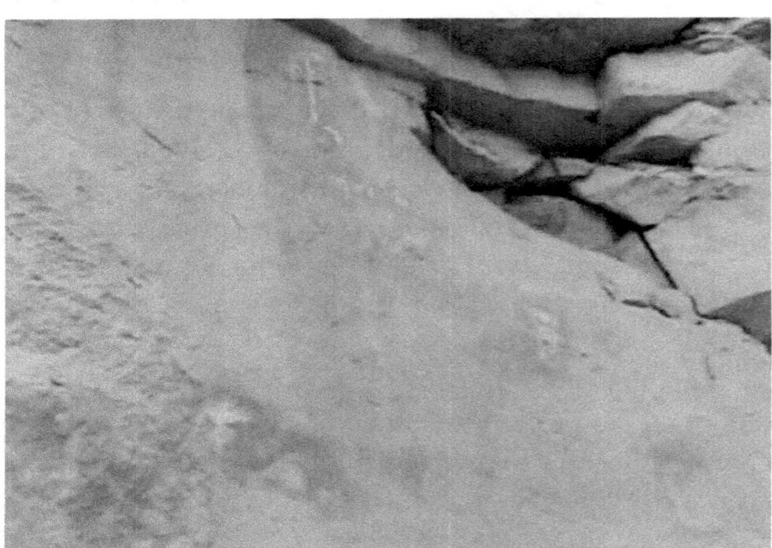

I held it there, hovering above the map, to see if I could get a "YES" from my pendulum over any portion of the map. I waited.

YES!

I was to go to the hieroglyph rocks! That required me to drive for a bit to get closer and then take about a mile walk in to reach the hieroglyphs. It was a warm October day, and I was glad I had brought plenty of water. I picked up the drum and the horn and the camera and started off onto the trail to the rocks. When I found the hieroglyphs, I set the camera on a rock and started filming myself. I sat down on a nearby rock and started to play my seven-chakra drum. I was calling the ancestors and asking for help with this task. There was a storm brewing in the distance to my left that stayed just far enough away that I had time to do the work. After playing my drum for a while, I took out my horn and started playing harmonics which are the complex chords created when you play and sing into the horn at the same time. It sounded otherworldly and fit perfectly into the space.

I had long understood that sound could create a space within which alignment was possible. All I had to do was create the space with my music and drumming. When I finished playing the horn, I started to chant and sing. At one point, I got up and went over to the rock wall on which the hieroglyphs were carved and sang harmonics into a crack in the rock. After about an hour I knew the camera was about to stop recording and I had done everything I could think of to do. I was unsure if I had accomplished my mission until I was packing up the camera.

I was doing one last pan of the area to my left. Something told me – and it wasn't so much a voice as it was a prodding feeling – to pan to the right. I took the camera off my eye and looked over to my right and saw nothing worthy of recording, but I aimed the camera to the right and started recording. There it was! I couldn't see it with my eyes, but the camera was recording it!

There was a beam of crystal white light shooting up from the Earth into the sky!

I was amazed and awed. I took away the camera and again looked with my eyes at the same area I was recording, but I saw nothing. But the camera was recording it! It was plain as day, a crystal beam of light shooting out of the Earth and up into the clouds.

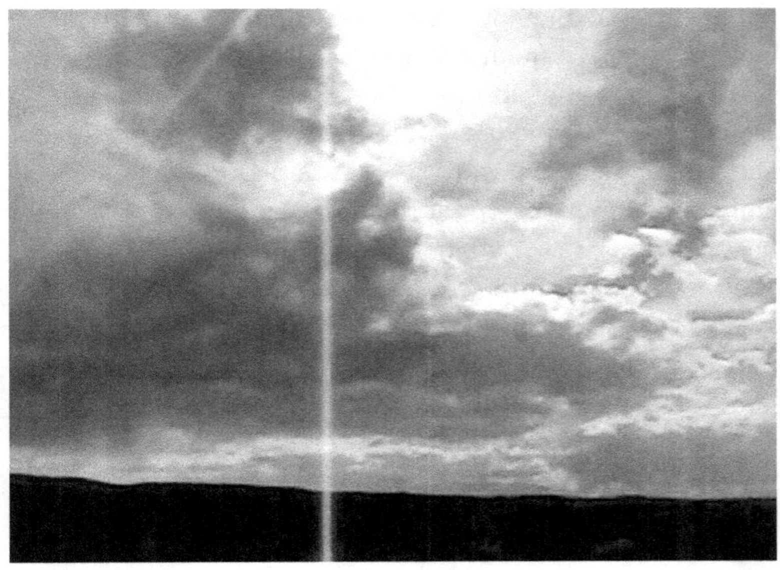

When I got back to Santa Fe, I uploaded the video to You-Tube and titled it Chaco *Canyon- Activating the Earth's Crystal Grid*. It's still there if you want to see it.

This is the description of the video on YouTube:

10/2/2011 to assist in the reactivation of the crystal grid network within the Earth that had been disabled with the destruction of Atlantis. After playing and singing harmonics, with the help of the ancestors and beings of light who assisted you will see a beam of light coming from the Earth shooting up into the sky. This crystal Earth network connects with the Net of Light which surrounds the planet, triangulates Earth's crystal pathways with the net of light pathways, and activates the 3rd strand of DNA within the planet and us to assist us with our expansion into our new 5th-dimensional awareness. (Dolores Cannon, New Earth)

This whole process was a miracle – the meditating, listening, and trusting my silently felt intuitions enough to follow through. I was humbled and very satisfied that I was able to accomplish my part of the overall project.

I showed the picture to my cousin, John, an Art Gallery Manager in Santa Fe who started as a photographer. He examined the photo and confirmed that it didn't look like the beam of light was coming out of the clouds and that it indeed was coming up from the Earth.

Miracle Story #4 – The Void

The Breath Pulse is a concept that was taught to me by my friend, Jim. It's a meditation that uses the breath to open a door to the dimension of Oneness. He demonstrated it to me several times and even sent me a recording of him demonstrating it. He used it as a technique to connect with the essence of another person and then he would sing them a blessing of sorts that always elevated and delighted them. It's a very good Oneness meditation that helps you to get to that third ingredient of a miracle that I call Oneness or Divinity.

The Breath Pulse is done with one breath. It starts on the sound "Ho" only made with the breath – no vocal cords – which symbolizes the masculine element of the 3rd-dimension. Then, in the same breath, you move to a "Ha" which symbolizes the feminine within the 3rd-dimension. Then, still in the same breath, you make the sound "Chi" – the life force energy – again with no vocalizing, just the breath and the mouth and tongue. At this point, you stop the sound for a short time to get ready to blast out of the 3rd-dimension and you enter the 2nd dimension with the exploding of the sound, "Tao" which you then blend into a "Hu" sound of ONE-NESS. On the "Hu", the breath and the shape of the lips form-ing the "Hu" vowel sound creates a type of whistling sound that carries you into ONENESS. The breath pules Ho, Ha, Chi, Tao, Hu moves you from the 3rd- dimension to the 2nd-di-mension and into oneness, which I experienced as the VOID in this particular miracle.

One evening, I had an unexpected allergic reaction to something I ate. At first, the allergic reaction started out as an itch, but over the course of an hour or two, it turned into an all-out hives attack with large blotches all over me that were more than itchy. I tried scratching, no help, I tried anti-itch cortisol cream, no help. I wished I had some Benadryl, but no luck. I went to bed hoping to get to sleep but that was impossible because of all the itching. Then I remem-bered how Jim told me he cured his prostate cancer. He said he spent so much time out of his body in the void in the con-sciousness of Oneness, that the cancer had nothing with which to connect. Jim's ego had melted into Oneness and the cancer no longer had a space in which to live.

That made sense to me, but I could not simply *will* myself out of my body. I had never had an out of body experience, except for one brief moment at the end of a dream when I saw myself moving through outer space towards the Earth and then waking up in my bed astonished at what I had just experienced. The only other way I knew of to get out of my body was to use the breath pulse. I had tried to do this at other times but had no luck. This time I was really desperate.

I realized I had an opportunity to surrender to the itch and allow myself to be vulnerable and open- hearted. I also had a very high emotional frequency, a very intense need.

As I was getting ready to receive a miracle in the space of Oneness. So, I began with that intention and with the understanding that I was asking for help. I took a deep breath and started the slow, soft chant:

Ho, Ha, Chi / TAO Huuuuuuu
(big breath)
Ho, Ha, Chi / TAO Huuuuuuu

As I chanted, I heard in myself that the Ho, even though I was not using my vocal cords, created a note inside my mouth, a harmonic of the breath. When I moved to the Ha from the Ho, the breath notes went up a major 3rd and moved from "do" to "mi". Then the Chi sound moved up to the "sol" just with the breath, no vocal cords. TAO had no pitch that I could discern, but the Hu sound that turned into a soft kind of whistle was an unrelated note that was lower than the Ho with which I started.

I had meditated for so long with the harmonic chords using my horn and trying to follow the harmonics off into the other dimensions, but I had never quite landed there. That night, it was as if the harmonics had moved me through the 3rd dimension into the duality of TAO (Ying, Yang) and then to Oneness. I actually heard a sound like a bubble popping while I felt my head gently breaking through some etheric barrier, and I ended up in the VOID. There was no sound. There was no light, there was just nothingness, complete stillness, and emptiness that felt full of potential. I lingered there for about five minutes, letting go of ego and blending into this Oneness, and then I popped back into my body.

The itching was completely gone. The hive patches were gone. The allergic reaction stopped dead in its tracks. I was okay again. Whatever had caused my body to react was suddenly moot, nonexistent, and my energy field had returned to its perfection.

Chapter 11

Your Personal Chakra Scale

You Are Music, Sing Your Body

As a musician and music lover, I am more kinesthetic than visual. That is, my primary senses with which I experience the world are hearing and touching as opposed to seeing and thinking. I find I can quiet my mind very quickly by using humming and sound during meditation as opposed to just sitting in silence. It's all about what makes sense to you. For me, I started meditation by playing long tones on my horn while singing into it at the same time. This created harmonic chords. As I asked my brain to hear all of the notes that were sounding in the chords, my mind shut down because the task was too formidable. It was a quick way to become still and calm.

That is what worked for me.

What will work for you? Combining meditation with something else that you love may give you the incentive to meditate every day. Find something that you enjoy doing and want to do every day that you can combine with meditation. You can meditate while you are walking, running, drawing, breathing, dancing, etc. If you pair meditation with doing something you love, then your motivation for meditating will increase exponentially.

Making harmonic chords on my horn was already very fulfilling for me, **and then I tried humming.**

If you keep your mouth closed, like you do while humming, the sound vibrations stay inside your body. It was while humming that I realized our bones could conduct the sounds to all parts of the body, especially if you're singing the right notes that correlate to the parts of your body. When I hummed the lowest note that I could comfortably hum, I felt a tingling sensation in my root chakra. It was like magic. That chakra that I had imagined for years but never *experienced as real* became palpable and tangible. My root chakra was not just a figment of my imagination. It was **real**! It existed in a physical place in my body, not my imagination.

Learning how to sing your root chakra is the first step to finding the notes to all of your chakras.

Why Knowing Your Chakra Scale is Helpful

Your chakra energy wheels connect to your glandular system. Once you know your chakra notes, you can energize the glands of your endocrine system.

Root = Adrenal glands make adrenaline, noradrenaline, and cortisol

Sacral = Ovaries, Gonads make testosterone and estrogen

Solar Plexus = Pancreas Gland makes insulin, glucagon, and gastrin

Heart = Thymus Gland makes thymosin (T cells)

Throat = Thyroid Gland makes T3 and T4

Third Eye = Pituitary Gland makes TSH, Oxytocin, and ACTH

Crown = Pineal Gland makes melatonin

These are not your grandfather's chakra imaginings.

I come to this endeavor from a very different perspective than a Yoga Master or a Meditation Master. I am a Sound Master. I am not going to ask you to imagine your chakras. I am going to help you feel your chakras vibrating with a sound that you make with your voice. I am going to help you hum. Feeling your chakra centers will help you begin a relationship with these now very tangible energy centers. When you hum your chakras, you will experience cause and effect through your voice and your sensations. It takes chakra meditations and clearings to the next level and helps to integrate their usefulness into your consciousness on a very practical, physical level as well as on an emotional, mental, and spiritual level.

I see chakras as our body's *Emotional Energy Cellular Distribution System.*

If you are fearful for your life and are in fight or flight mode, then the fear emotion tells your brain to make more adrenaline so that you can run faster and survive whatever it is that is making you run for your life. When fear triggers our fight or flight response, an entire biochemical cascade of hormones like adrenalin and cortisol are released. These hormones increase heart rate, slow digestion, push blood flow to major muscle groups, and adjust various other autonomic nervous functions that give the body a burst of energy and strength. Then, when you are out of danger, the relief emotion tells your brain to make more nor- adrenaline which stops all the adrenaline and cortisol and so on.

The point is that our *emotions* turn hormones on and off. Emotions live in our emotional etheric energy space about three or four inches out from the body. Emotional energy/frequency is literally distributed into our cells.

Chakras are etherically connected to major glands that produce hormones that regulate metabolism, fight or flight response, bone and tissue growth, sexual functions, bonding, blood pressure, immune system, waking up, falling asleep, and more. Once you know your personal chakra notes, you begin to have some control over these systems by humming and listening to your notes since humming your chakras activates your Emotional Energy Cellular Distribution System. The chakras are like the hardware that the body uses to distribute its emotions into its cells.

Learning your body's personal chakra scale notes and your body's musical key will balance your emotions and calm your nerves for relief of Anxiety, PTSD, Insomnia, and Depression. You will experience firsthand your chakras actually vibrating because **the sound spectrum of our individual voices reveals the musical key to which our bodies are tuned**.

You don't have to believe anything I say about this. You will experience this vibrating yourself and you'll know it is true because of your firsthand, physical, tangible experience of it. The subtle vibration helps to release stuck cellular emotional memory from the cells of your body that could be causing you pain and sleepless nights. When strong emotional energy is not carefully processed at the time that it happens, it lies stagnant in our cells in a place in our body that is somehow connected to that same strong feeling.

As I said earlier, energy can't be destroyed or deleted, it can only be changed. That strong emotional energy that we didn't have time to process at the moment or that we didn't know how to process or that we didn't have the support we needed to process gets deposited somewhere in our body. It languishes and causes a disharmony that eventually becomes a kind of pain.

Our emotions, conscious or unconscious, owned or stuffed, are distributed into our cells by our chakras.

Have you ever had a nagging pain? Did you try everything under the sun to relieve it? Did something work for a while, but it kept coming back? If your pain was triggered by unconscious emotions, then physical remedies will not get to the root cause of the pain. It's really tough to get to the root cause of something that is unconscious! Sound frequencies can vibrate the cellular memory and release that old energy so your body can heal without having to talk about or relive the memory!

If a memory of a traumatic feeling gets stuck in our cellular memory, over time it could become dis-eased. That is why some aches and pains just keep coming back. If we have tried everything to heal a part of our body, and it only works for a while and then it comes back over and over again, it could be that the injury is rooted in an unconscious emotional memory. You can't fix something in the physical plane if it was initiated in the emotional plane.

Sound and vibration are processed with the most primitive part of our brains, not our pre-frontal lobe. We can't figure out with our logic a way to fix something that started as emotion and is now unconscious. If we buried it because we didn't know how to deal with it, we had to stuff it into a place where we wouldn't remember it. We all do this as part of our survival protocol.

When we vibrate our chakras with the proper frequency, it realigns that old cellular memory that is no longer serving us so that it vibrates more in harmony with our system. **The sound creates a space at the cellular level that allows for realignment.** Sound gets to the root of the problem and allows the body to adjust and heal from the emotional trauma without having to re-experience the memory in any way.

You may have feelings of sadness after you listen to the sounds. It doesn't mean that something is wrong with you. It means something needs to process in you. Just let the feelings flow through you. Have a cry if you need to have a cry. Your body is releasing old, unconscious, emotional cellular memory. Don't fight it, just let them release. Then you can send white light into the space that just released the feelings. The body will really like the white light.

The body would naturally try to bring back those familiar sad feelings again because it was used to having that vibration there. But when you present the body with the high-frequency white light, it greatly prefers it to the old feelings. It will help your healing last if you bring in the white light.

The conventional wisdom about the notes that correspond to the seven major chakra centers in your body is that a C major scale is best. Every book or chart that I could find dealing with the sounds of the chakras always displayed a C major scale. Like I mentioned before, all human beings *do not* naturally resonate to a C major scale but to a Lydian scale that starts with the note that is at the bottom of your vocal range.

We all have different vocal ranges. Some of us have very low voices, others have higher voices. Our root chakra note will depend on how low our voice can hum. This means we each have a different starting note for our Lydian scale.

The Lydian scale differs from the C major scale on only one note which happens to be the note that correlates to the heart chakra. In the C major scale, that note would be F, but that note doesn't vibrate the heart chakra; F sharp does (F#). The scale that vibrates all of the seven major chakras of human beings is a Lydian scale: Do, Re, Mi, **Fi**, Sol, La, Ti. Note the difference between this and the C major scale: Do, Re, Mi, **Fa**, Sol, La, Ti.

Some of us have Root chakras with the note D, and others are F or E flat. It all depends on the vocal range of the person. One woman, upon learning to vibrate her chakras after having tried to visualize them for years, was ecstatic. She said, "This is fabulous work. It's so real, it's so right, it's so the missing pieces!"

After working with many clients who were using their voices to find the notes that vibrated their chakras, I discovered that many people would settle on a note for a chakra that was in between the notes of the piano. They were feeling their chakras vibrate, but the note they were singing was in between the keys of the piano. This led me to believe that **human beings do not resonate with the A = 440 Hz scale**. There are recent studies that prove that the A = 432 Hz scale lowers heart rate, blood pressure, and anxiety. It has also been shown to repair DNA. This is the frequency to which my chimed mp3s are tuned.

How to Sing Your Root Chakra

1. It's sometimes easier to do this early in the morning when your voice is relaxed. It's best to be laying down on your back. Receive a deep breath and audibly sigh down to the lowest sound you can make. Do this three times. If you are trying this later in the day, this will loosen up your vocal cords in your low voice register.

2. Now close your mouth and hum down to the lowest sound you can comfortably make without straining your voice. This sound will not be a sound that you can project loudly, but it will be a sound that you can sustain. Once you think you have found it, hum it a few times using deep breaths so you can hum it for

at least ten seconds. If you have the right note, you will feel a slight vibration in your root chakra which is at the end of your spine near your coccyx or "sits" bone. It is a very subtle feeling. Some people describe it as a tingling sensation, others say they feel a slight pressure or warmth in the area of the chakra. If you don't feel anything at first, don't worry. This is a difficult chakra to feel because it is in a very dense part of our body. It usually takes a few repetitions to really feel it.

3. If you can't feel anything and you think you have the lowest note that you can comfortably sing, slowly hum upwards with your voice and notice where you *are* feeling the sounds in your body. You can start on the lowest note that you can comfortably sing and hum up the scale like Do, Re, Mi, Fa. When you get to "Fa" where do you feel that? If it's in your abdomen, hum up one note higher and you should feel your heart chakra vibrating. Your heart chakra and throat chakra are the easiest to feel. There is so much air in your lungs/heart chakra area, which makes that part of the body easy to vibrate. Note that your throat is vibrating on every note you sing, so that is not a good place to start. But, if you feel your heart chakra vibrating and then you hum up a half step to the next closest note, you will feel your throat chakra vibrate. Then you will know you have the right notes. You can use the chart below to find all the notes of your chakra scale once you have found either your root or heart chakra note.

I realize that you are probably not accustomed to feeling your voice move energy in your body. Once you learn to use your voice to direct energy to all parts of your body, you'll wonder why you were never taught this in school. It is such a natural thing to do. Our brains use the sound of our voices as biofeedback information all day long, whether we are aware of it or not.

Learning to consciously sing your body is very rewarding. It gives you a sense of dominion over your own health! As our voices reveal our weaknesses to the brain, we can listen to our bodies and hum back what we hear, thereby helping our bodies respond and repair themselves. Yes, we can listen for our Spontaneous Otto Acoustic Emissions in our ears, and the sound we hear will tell us exactly what the body needs at that moment.

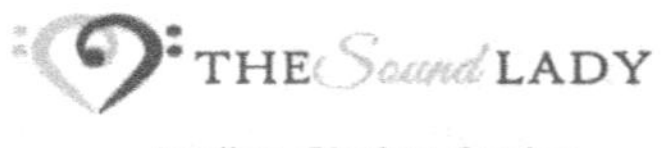

Lydian Chakra Scales

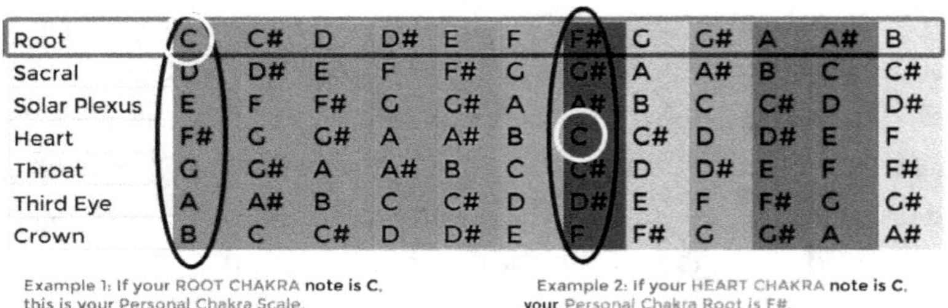

Root	C	C#	D	D#	E	F	F#	G	G#	A	A#	B
Sacral	D	D#	E	F	F#	G	G#	A	A#	B	C	C#
Solar Plexus	E	F	F#	G	G#	A	A#	B	C	C#	D	D#
Heart	F#	G	G#	A	A#	B	C	C#	D	D#	E	F
Throat	G	G#	A	A#	B	C	C#	D	D#	E	F	F#
Third Eye	A	A#	B	C	C#	D	D#	E	F	F#	G	G#
Crown	B	C	C#	D	D#	E	F	F#	G	G#	A	A#

Example 1: If your ROOT CHAKRA **note is C,** this is your Personal Chakra Scale.

Example 2: If your HEART CHAKRA **note is C,** your Personal Chakra Root is F#.

COPYRIGHT © THE SOUND LADY

When you know your chakra notes, it's possible to know which notes will vibrate other parts of your body that are near your chakras. For instance, if your Heart Chakra note is B and your Solar Plexus Chakra note is A, the note in between them will vibrate the parts of your body that are in be-tween those two chakra centers. Your liver is in between your Solar Plexus chakra and your Heart chakra, therefore the note A sharp will vibrate your liver and gallbladder and the organs of your stomach. If you have stuffy sinuses, the note for your sinus is going to be between the note for your Throat chakra and your Third Eye chakra because your sinuses are between your throat and your Third Eye. If you hum that note, you can begin to clear your sinuses.

Knowing your personal chakra notes begins to give you dominion over your health. They are a starting point for the health of your body parts. Humming your chakras will vibrate them where they attach to your physical body. This vibration is often sufficient to reset the energy back to neutral. The result of this is calm emotions and balanced hormones that are responsible for turning systems on and off.

In just a bit, we'll talk about the other stuff that gets vibrated besides your physical body, but for now, the **Your Body's Musical Key Chakra Note Pattern Chart** is how to vibrate other parts of your body that are close to the chakra centers. They are vibrated by a pitch that is close to the note of the nearest chakra center. Knowing your chakra scale is not only good for balancing emotions, but also for relieving pain. The vibration that the sound of your voice makes in your body brings oxygenation and circulation to the vibrating area. This oxygenation and circulation initiate your body's natural healing processes.

Your voice, carried on the breath, directed upward or downward through your choice of vowel sounds and your intention, brings your issue to the top of the brain's triage list and gets it off the back burner.

Humming like this gives the body energy to deal with an issue that it previously did not have the energy to deal with.

The chart below shows the in-between notes for other body parts if your Root chakra is the note F, for example.

Your Body's Musical Key
Chakra Note Pattern Chart

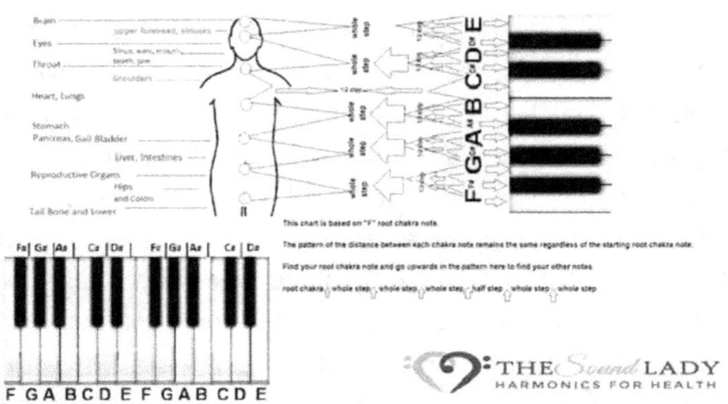

To find your in-between notes for your other body parts, first, find the chakra that is below the body part you want to oxygenate and vibrate. Let's say you want to work on your ears or eustachian tubes because they are clogged. The chakra below that part of your body is your Throat chakra, let's say your Throat chakra note is A. Use the chart below to find the note that is one half-step above the note A. Note that the sharp notes (#) raise the natural note one half-step higher than the note below it. In this case, your ear and eustachian tubes note would be A sharp. Humming that note for ten minutes will help to drain your Eustachian tubes of fluid.

Or if your sinuses are stuffy, follow the same process as for the Eustachian tubes. The sinuses are located between the Throat and Third Eye chakras. If your Throat chakra is E and your Third Eye chakra is F sharp, then your sinuses, ears, jaw, teeth, gums, and tongue will vibrate physically to the note in between those two chakra notes – F. Humming the note F for ten minutes will begin to drain your sinuses, ears, gums.

There is one whole step in between all the major chakras except for between the Heart and Throat chakras where there is only one half-step.

One whole step consists of two half-steps. These steps are how the space between two notes is measured. The smallest distance between two notes in Western music is a half-step. Since there is a whole step between all of the chakras except between the Heart and Throat chakras, it is not hard to find the in-between notes. There is always a note in between each chakra (except for between the Heart and the Throat) and it is a half-step above the lower chakra.

On the keyboard below, there is a half-step or semitone in between each note – white or black. There is a semitone in between the first white note on this keyboard – F – and the black note next to it – F sharp. Between the black note – F sharp – and the next higher white note – G – is also a half-step. There is a whole step between the notes F and G.

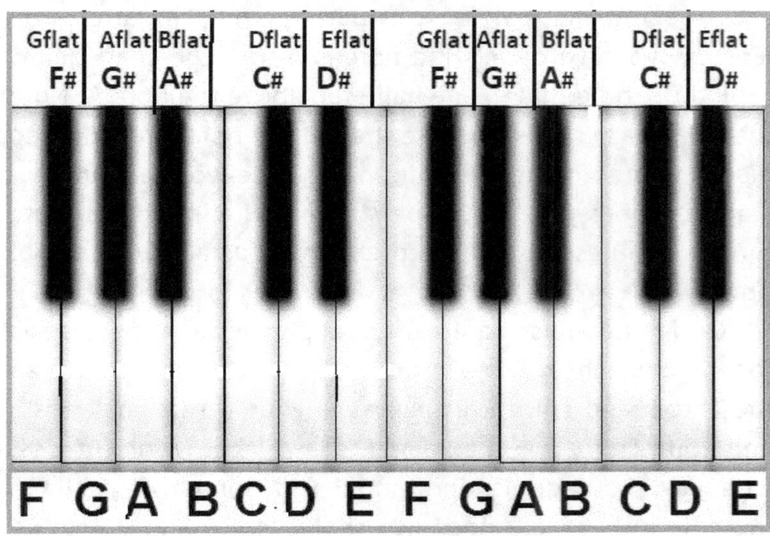

The white keys go from left to right in the order of the alphabet. Notes are named ABCDEFG then they repeat in the next octave- ABCDEFG etc.

Notice that each black key has 2 different note names. ie F# is the same note as Gflat, G# is the same note as Aflat ect.

When there is a black key between 2 white keys, it means that there is a whole step between those 2 notes.

When there is no black key in between 2 white keys it means there is a ½ step between those 2 notes.

Since there is already only a semitone in between the Throat and Heart chakras, we have to find the note that vibrates the space in between the Heart and Throat chakras a bit differently. One way to find a vibration that is smaller than a semitone is to play the two notes for the Throat chakra and Heart chakra simultaneously. On a pitch pipe, there is a semitone in between each blowhole. If your Heart chakra note is D and your Throat Chakra note is D sharp, then those two blowholes are right next to each other on the pitch pipe. You can blow into both of the holes at the same time. The combination of two semitones creates a harmonic that is half the distance between those two notes.

The Aura and Human Magnetic Field

When we work with the energy of our chakras, we are working with our aura which is also known as our magnetic field or biofield. Our magnetic field surrounds and intertwines with our physical body and is shaped like a torus. This is a geometric shape that seems to naturally repeat its pattern in everything from the tiniest of atoms to the enormity of galaxies. Foster Gamble is an author and producer of the film, *Thrive: What on Earth Will It Take?* He explains, "Looking back on almost half a century of research, including thousands of books, films, interviews with experts from diverse fields, if I were to pick one common denominator to all the facets of my quest, it would be the TORUS, the fundamental energy pattern that invites our alignment at every level of our existence for us to survive and thrive."

The torus is a donut-shaped geometric pattern of energy movement. It has a continuous surface with a hole in it where the energy moves in from one end, circulates around the center, and then exits out the other end.

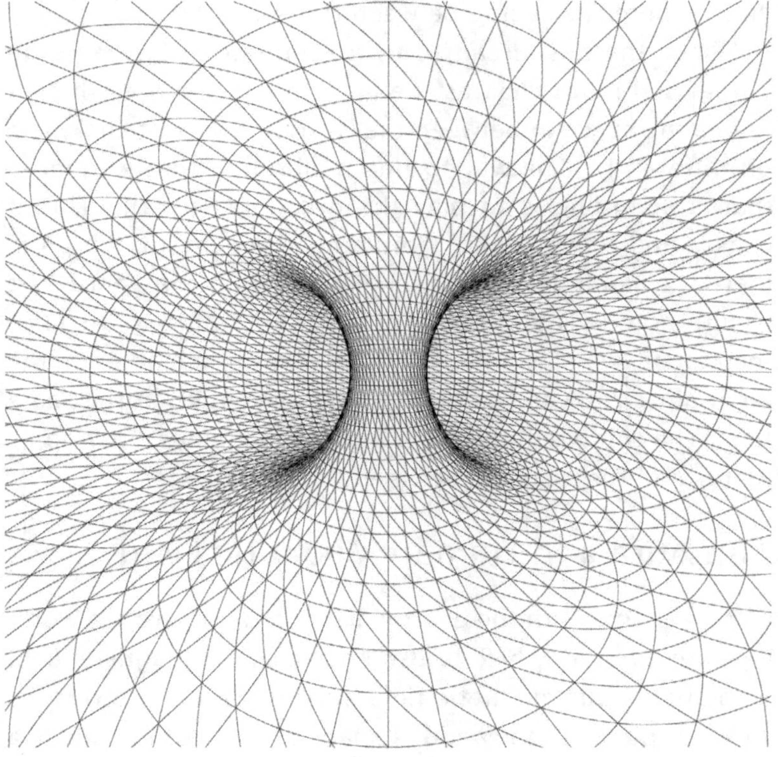

It is the only energy pattern that can sustain itself. Humans have a toroidal energy shape. We have a hole down our center from mouth to intestinal tract, and our skin is the continuous surface. The Earth, trees, shells, and the galaxy are all examples of the toroidal energy pattern.

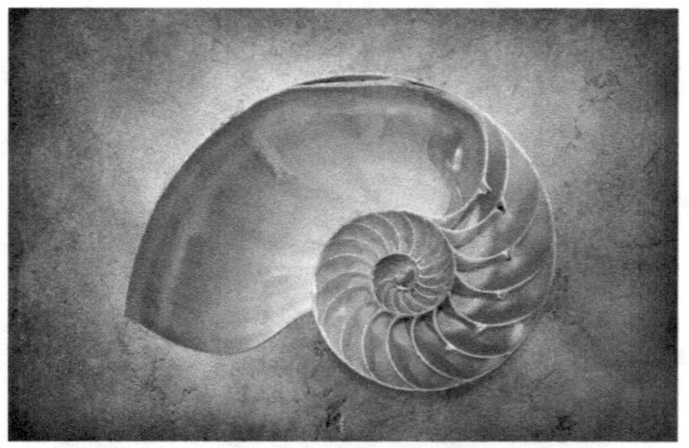

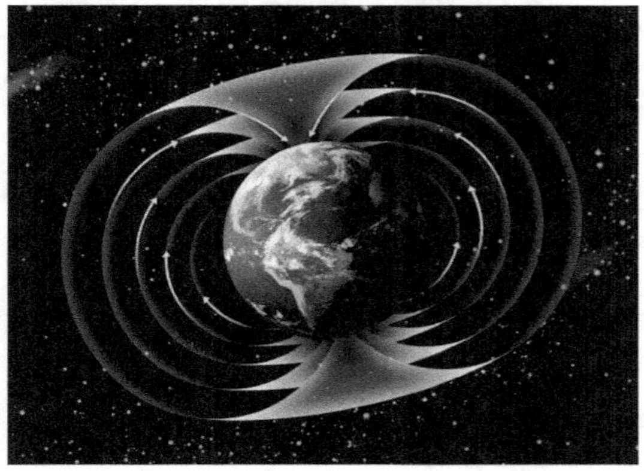

This magnetic field is both uniquely ours and also connected to everything else as it is made out of the same substance as its surroundings. When we work with our chakras, we are working with this central column of energy that is the hole in the donut shape where energy enters and exits.

Chapter 12

Your Personal Chakra Scale Guided Meditation

You can use a pitch pipe (chromatic C to C) for this guided meditation, or you can hum along with the Personal Chakra Scale with Guided Meditation mp3 for your body's musical key. This can be purchased and downloaded from **www.the-soundlady.com** as a private session.

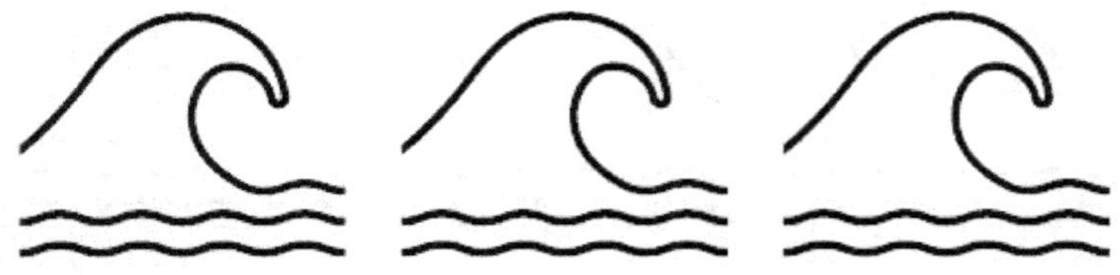

Breathing through your nose, receive a breath. Exhale through your mouth and pause.

Breath in through your nose again. Hold the air in your lungs. Hug it gratefully with your ribs.

Exhale love and thankfulness to the consciousness of the Breath and pause as the sound of the breath goes into the void where all sound originates. Then, receive another breath.

*As you listen to or blow your **Root chakra** note on the pitch pipe, imagine the color red and know that you are a survivor.*

Inhale again, and hum or blow on the pitch pipe the note of your root chakra three times.

This time, as you inhale and begin to hum your root chakra note, let the hum move to the front of the mouth. Slowly open your lips and let out a "muh" sound to fill the room.

Imagine the room is filling with the color red and the sound of your chakra. Then, close your lips and bring the sound and color back inside yourself.

Relax now for a minute or two while this sound assimilates into your system. If you are humming along with the chimes mp3, breathe gratefully and let the sound settle into your body.

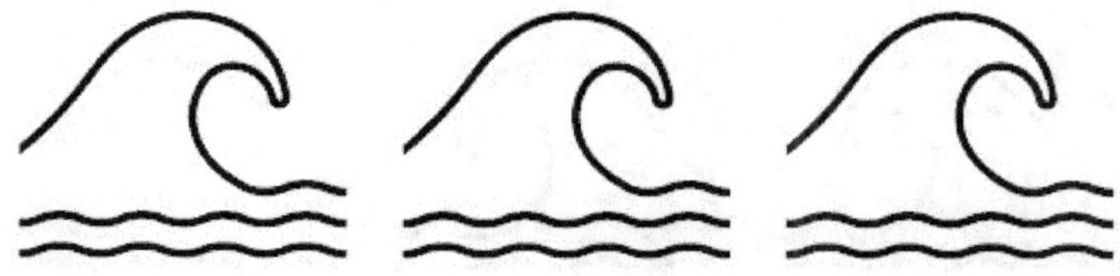

*As you listen, hum, or play your **Sacral chakra** note, inhale the sound of it into your Sacral chakra.*

Honoring all others and imagining the color orange, hum or blow your Sacral chakra note three times.

Inhale again, and let the hum move to the front of the mouth. Slowly open your lips and let out a "moh" sound to fill the room.

Imagine the room is filling with the color orange and the sound of your chakra. Then, close your lips and bring the sound and color back inside yourself.

Relax now for a minute or two while this sound assimilates into your system. If you are humming along with the mp3, breathe gratefully and let the sound settle into your body.

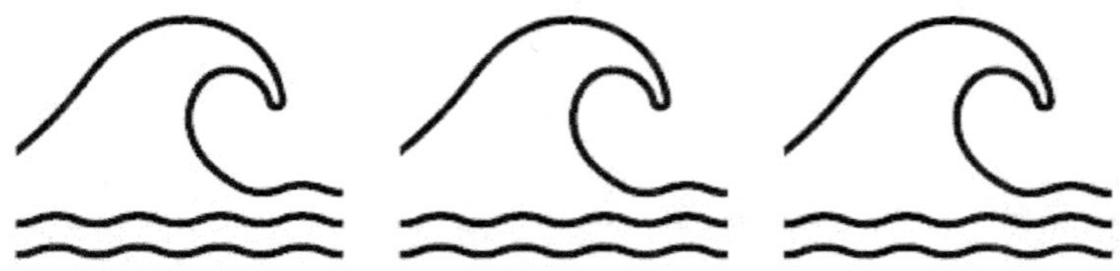

*Next, inhale your **Solar Plexus chakra** note into your Solar Plexus chakra. Imagine the color yellow and feel it amplifying your will power.*

Listen to, hum, or play your Solar Plexus chakra note three times.

Inhale again and let the hum move to the front of the mouth. Slowly open your lips and let out a "moo" sound to fill the room.

Imagine the room is filling with the color yellow and the sound of your chakra. Then, close your lips and bring the sound and color back inside.

Relax now for a minute or two while this sound assimilates into your system. If you are humming along with the mp3, breathe gratefully and let the sound settle into your body while you listen to the ocean waves.

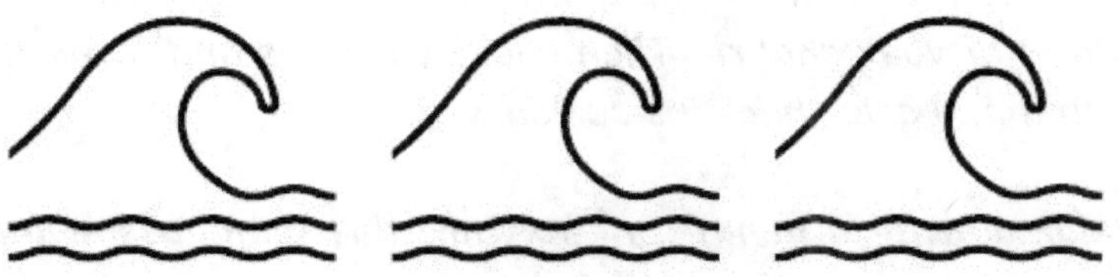

*Now, inhale your **Heart chakra** note into your Heart chakra. Imagine the color green and feel your compassion expanding.*

Listen to, hum, or play your Heart chakra note three times. Inhale again and let the hum move to the front of the mouth. Slowly open your lips and let out a "mah" sound to fill the room.

Imagine the room is filling with the color green and the sound of your chakra. Then, close your lips and bring the sound and color back inside yourself.

Relax now for a minute or two while this sound assimilates into your system. If you are humming along with the mp3, breathe gratefully and let the sound settle into your body while you listen to the ocean waves.

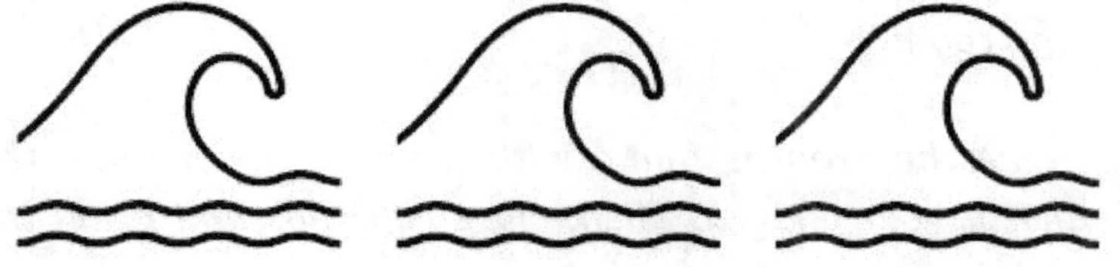

*Now, inhale your **Throat chakra** note into your Throat chakra. Imagine the color blue and know you are speaking your truth.*

Listen to, hum, or play your Throat chakra note three times.

On the last chime for this chakra, let the sound move to the front of your mouth. Slowly open your lips and let out a "may" sound to fill the room.

Imagine the room filling with the color blue, and then close your lips and bring the sound and color back inside.

Relax now for a minute or two while this sound assimilates into your system. If you are humming along with the mp3, breathe gratefully and let the sound settle into your body while you listen to the ocean waves.

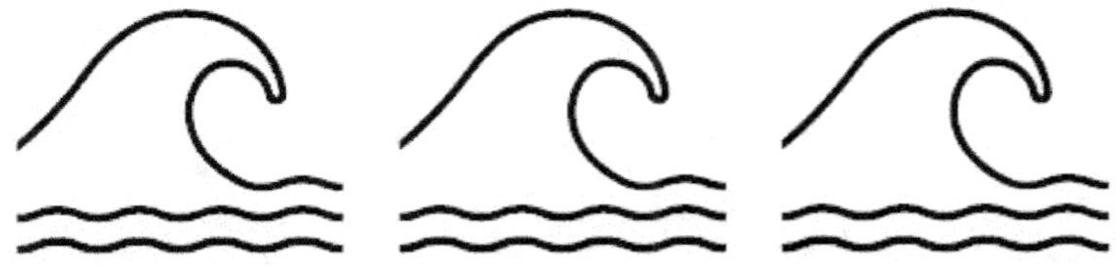

*Inhale your **Third Eye chakra note** into your Third Eye. Imagine the color purple enhancing your inner vision.*

Listen to, hum, or play your Third Eye chakra note three times.

On the last chime for this chakra, let the sound move to the front of your mouth. Slowly open your lips and let out a "mee" sound to fill the room.

Imagine the room filling with the color purple and the sound of your chakra. Then, close your lips and bring the sound and color back inside.

Relax now for a minute or two while this sound assimilates into your system. If you are humming along with the mp3, breathe gratefully and let the sound settle into your body while you listen to the ocean waves.

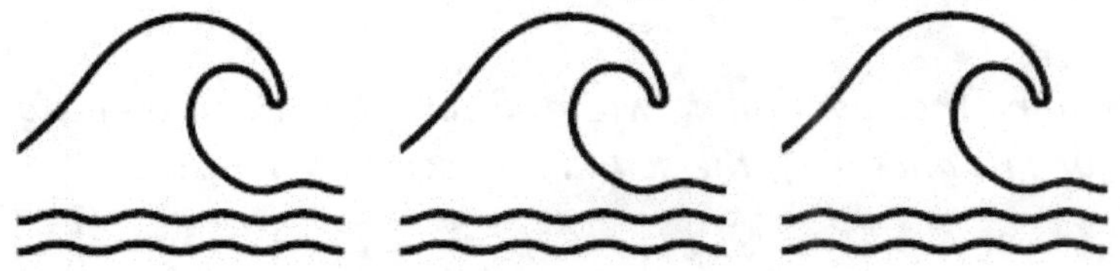

Inhale your **Crown chakra note** into your Crown chakra. Imagine the color white and remember to be mindful.

Listen to, hum, or your Crown chakra note three times.

On the next chime, make the sound "wooooosh" as you exhale.

Relax now for a minute or two while this sound assimilates into your system. If you are humming along with the mp3, breathe gratefully and let the sound settle into your body while you listen to the ocean waves.

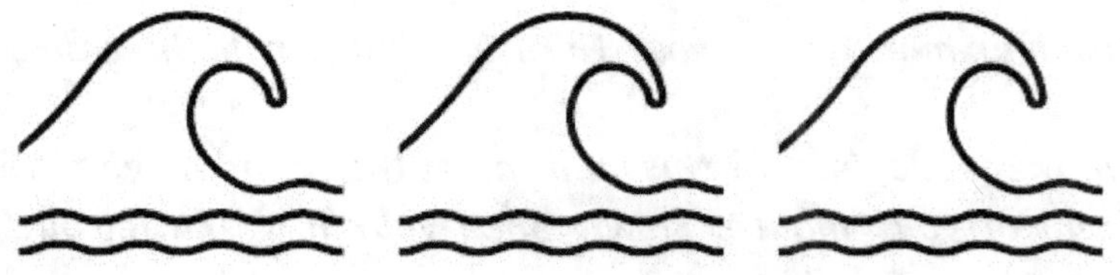

Starting with the Crown chakra, hum each chakra note once with the chimes to bring your energy back down to your root chakra.

Relax in the stillness and calm for several minutes to let the vibrations assimilate with your energy field.

Chapter 13

Connect All Chakras Through the Heart

Infinity Loop Meditation

Once you have energized your chakras by singing/humming them, there is a way to connect them for maximum energy flow. Everything connects through the heart. The heart is the junction box for the rest of the chakras. When you use the infinity loop visualization to connect the lower chakras to the higher chakras through the heart, you are energizing your biofield or auric field or electromagnetic field. Your biofield is your body's protection from harmful or negative energies that you may encounter day to day out in the world. It's a wonderful practice to get back to your home state of being while you listen to or hum along with your personal chakra scale. It resets your emotional state back to neutral and removes dissonance from your field that got stuck to you out in the world.

An infinity loop is a mathematical symbol. It represents limitlessness or eternity. It has had many meanings to different cultures throughout time. Going back to the 5th Century AD, a Greek philosopher, Proclus, saw that the cross-sections of the torus created this infinity shape.

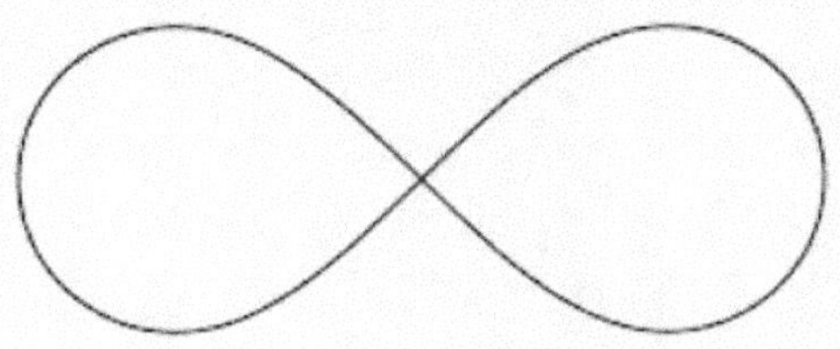

As it relates to the torus, it is the inner moving energy part of this self- sustaining energy field. It is why I use this shape to connect the lower chakras to the higher chakras through the intersection of the heart.

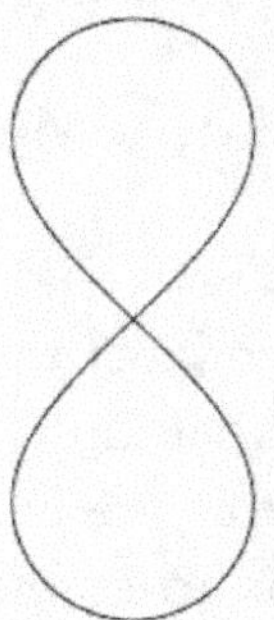

To connect all the chakras through the heart center, which is the junction box of the body's energy, use these three triads or three-note chords:

First Triad – The Root connects to the Heart and Crown chakras via the infinity loop energy pattern.

Second Triad – The Sacral chakra connects through the Heart to the Third Eye chakra.

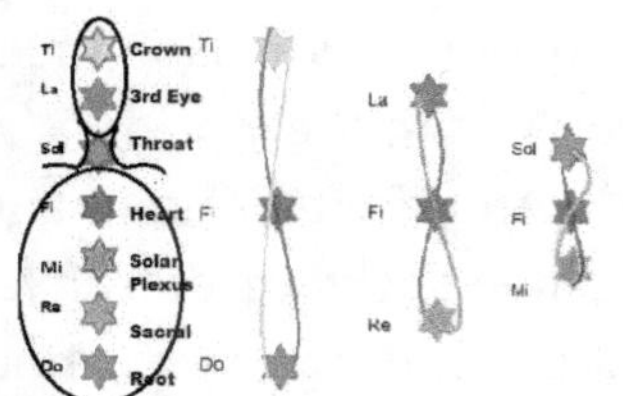

Third Triad – The Solar Plexus chakra connects through the Heart to the Throat chakra.

By using this imagery, we can energize the toroidal energy field that surrounds and permeates us. Imagine an infinity loop connecting Root and Crown chakras through the Heart while humming your Root, Heart, and Crown chakra notes up and down.

If your Root chakra note is C, then your first triad of chords that will connect your Root chakra to Crown chakra through the Heart chakra are the notes C, F sharp, and B. These notes are on the upward path of the infinity wave. On the downward path of the infinity wave, the notes are B, F sharp, and C.

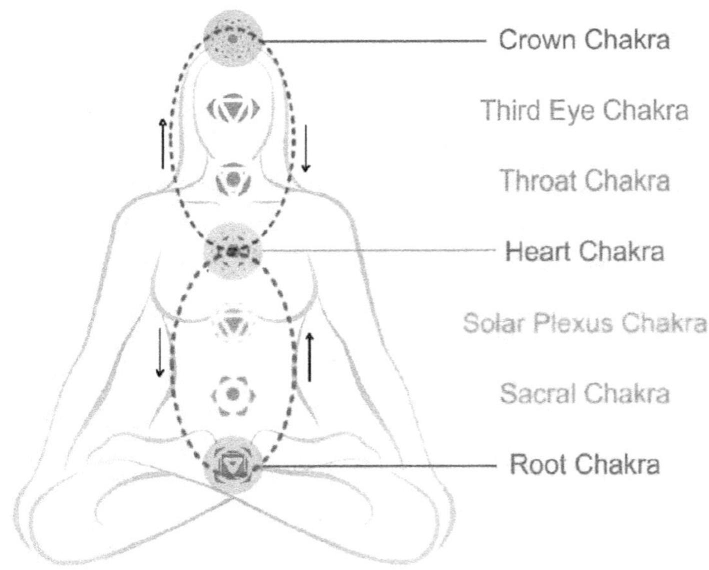

Your second triad would connect your Sacral chakra to your Third Eye chakra through your Heart. The upward notes would be D, F sharp, A, and the downward notes would be A, F sharp, D.

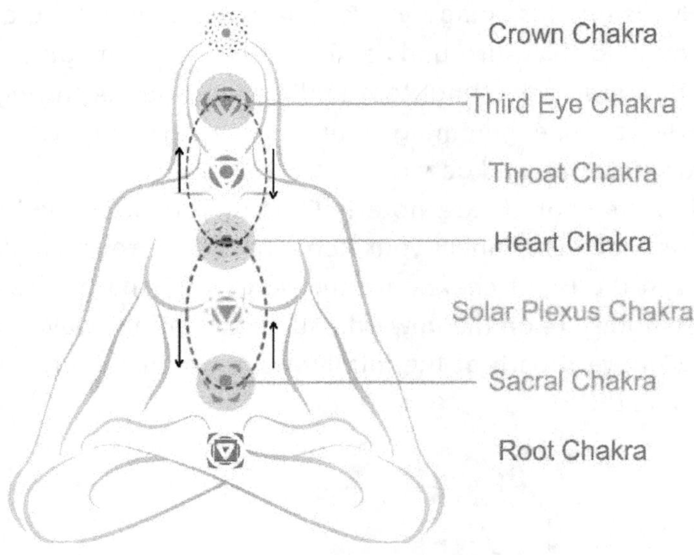

Your third triad infinity loop would connect your Solar Plexus chakra to your Throat chakra through your Heart. The upward notes of the infinity wave would be E, F sharp, G, and the downward notes would be G, F sharp, E.

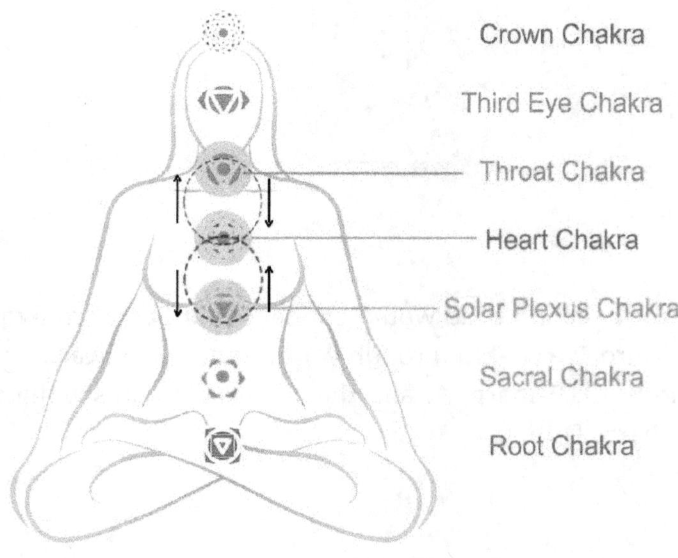

Connect Charkas Through the Heart
Guided Meditation

*Connect your **Root and Crown** chakras through the Heart chakra by humming or playing this combination three times:*

Root note, Heart note, Crown note, Heart note, Root note.

As you hum these notes, concentrate on moving the energy up your body with your voice. Visualize the energy moving in the shape of an infinity loop with the Heart at the center of the loop. Feel your voice pulling the energy upwards and then downwards back toward the Root.

Sing these three notes three more times while you:

Imagine your Root chakra energy of survival being informed with the compassion of your Heart.

Imagine the compassion of your Heart chakra energy informing your Crown chakra.

Feel your Crown chakra energy of higher wisdom informing your Heart's Compassion.

Merge the Root chakra and Crown chakra energy with your Heart energy.

*Connect your **Sacral and Third Eye** chakras through the Heart chakra by humming or playing this combination three times:*

Sacral note, Heart note, Third Eye note, Heart note, Sacral note.

As you hum these notes, concentrate on moving the energy up your body with your voice. Visualize the energy moving in the shape of an infinity loop with the Heart at the center of the loop. Feel your voice pulling the energy upwards and then downwards back toward the Sacral chakra.

Sing these three notes three more times while you:

Imagine your Sacral chakra energy of creativity being informed with the compassion of your Heart.

Imagine the compassion of your Heart chakra energy informing your Third Eye chakra.

Feel your Third Eye chakra energy of inner wisdom informing your Heart's Compassion.

Merge the Sacral chakra and Third Eye chakra energy with your Heart energy.

*Connect your **Solar Plexus and Throat** chakras through the Heart chakra by humming or playing this combination three times:*

Solar Plexus note, Heart note, Throat note, Heart note, Solar Plexus note.

As you hum these notes, concentrate on moving the energy up your body with your voice. Visualize the energy moving in the shape of an infinity loop with the Heart at the center of the loop. Feel your voice pulling the energy upwards and then downwards back toward the Solar Plexus chakra. Sing these three notes three more times while you:

Imagine your Solar Plexus chakra energy of creativity being informed with the compassion of your Heart.

Imagine the compassion of your Heart chakra energy in-forming your Throat chakra.

Feel your Throat chakra energy of communicating your truth informing your Heart's Compassion.

Merge the Solar Plexus chakra and Throat chakra energy with your Heart energy.

Humming the notes of your personal chakra scale while listening along with your personal chakra scale chimes mp3 and then humming your chakra connections through the heart infinity loops will ground you, center you, and leave you in an open-hearted state of being.

Chapter 14

Harmonics Are
Full-Spectrum Sound

Presenting the brain with a harmonic chord is like giving it a buffet of nutritious sounds to work with and feed on.

Harmonics are full-spectrum sound. It's easier to understand harmonics if you think of them as full-spectrum colors similar to full- spectrum light. When one note is played, depending on the resonance of the room, the more harmonics in that note, the fuller the sound. The harmonics of a note are the brother and sister tones that sound along with the main note because they are mathematically related. It's a natural phenomenon of the physics of sound; it's how a sound naturally expands.

Sound expands like cells divide. One becomes two becomes four becomes eight becomes sixteen and so on. The more harmonics that are sounding, the bigger and fuller the sound.

Given that the brain is a frequency monitor, it understands the physics of how sound expands. When the brain hears a harmonic chord, it understands the pattern. Presenting the brain with a harmonic chord is like inviting it to a buffet where it can pick and choose from the recognized pattern which notes it needs to create balance.

Harmonics are the result of the natural expansion of sustained sounds in a resonant environment.

Harmonics are the notes that naturally sound together with the main note if the sound is sustained long enough in a resonant environment. Harmonics sound along with the main note because they are mathematically related and have sound waves that resonate sympathetically with the main note. The more harmonics that are sounding within the note make the note sound fuller and richer. Harmonics are a result of the phenomenon of the physics of sound called The Harmonic Series of Notes. Here are the first 20 harmonics of the note C:

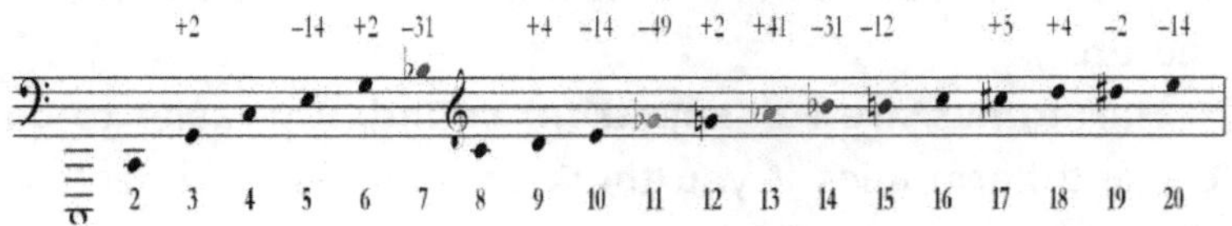

The Harmonic Series is the predictable series of notes which expand from a sustained sound. The harmonics are integer multiples of the fundamental: 1/2, 1/3, 1/4, 1/5, 1/6, etc.

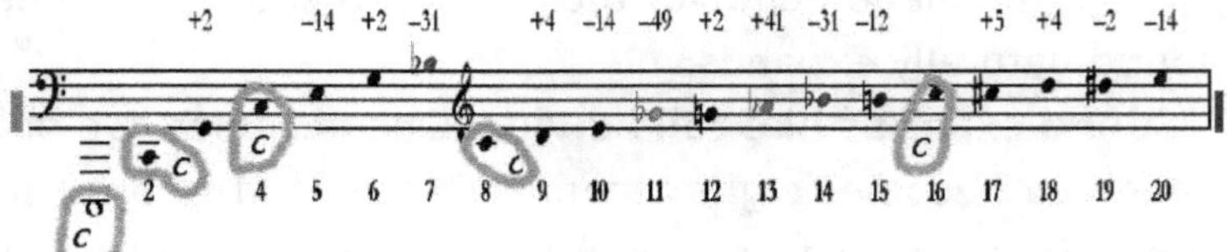

Of the first 20 harmonics, the note C sounds five times in five different octaves. As the C sound expands, some of its harmonics are louder than others – the octaves – because they are mathematically the most closely related to the fundamental. Their wavelengths vibrate most sympathetically with the fundamental, and they amplify the original note. This means that whenever a frequency doubles in speed, its sound is an octave higher.

You can also make harmonics when you play two notes at the same time. Two notes sounding at the same time can create a harmony that also produces harmonics from the sound waves of the two main notes.

This predictable progression of an expanding sound, the phenomenon called The Harmonic Series of Notes, is easily recognized by the brain. The brain is a frequency receiver and transmitter; it understands the physics of sound. The brain knows how sound expands and can readily use these frequencies to trigger the body's natural healing abilities. Harmonics are a predictable set of notes that always expand out of a fundamental – the main note you are sounding.

The brain knows this pattern of predictable notes like it knows the back of your hand.

Chapter 15

Chakra Harmonics

Creating Harmonics with the
Voice & Lips

Voice

Different vowel sounds create different harmonics. Inhale and sing the vowel sound "oooo" on any pitch that is comfortable for you. While staying on the same pitch, slowly change to the vowel sound "eeee." You will hear different harmonics with each vowel sound. As in the study with the aura cameras, harmonics are an important tool for talking to the brain in its language. The brain is fluent in the language of frequency.

Another good harmonic to try is singing any pitch you like using the vowel sound "EEEE" and changing to an "RRRR" while staying on the same pitch. Then change back to "EEEE" while still remaining on the same pitch. This will produce harmonics.

Lip Buzzing

Making buzzing sounds with your lips is another type of toning that can create harmonics for the brain to utilize. When I was a child, I used to make buzzing sounds with my lips because it made them feel funny and made me giggle. Blowing "raspberries" is just plain fun. Try it!

Take a deep breath in, and blow air out of your mouth with your lips pursed together causing them to flap. Try to sustain this for ten seconds. Note: laughter may ensue, so enjoy the playfulness of this sound!

Repeat the above step, but this time as you flap your lips, hum a pitch and sustain it for as long as you can. To begin, try ten seconds.

Take a deep breath and purse your lips together more tightly so that when you blow you create a pitch that you can sustain for ten seconds.

After mastering that last step, you can then add humming a different pitch to the one you are blowing.

This will create very rewarding harmonics that will make you tingle all over. Your brain will be floating in synovial fluid which is vibrating and massaging the brain. When you buzz and hum, it is a very gratifying feeling. It's like getting high, but it's legal and FREE!

Chakra Harmonics

To get to the root of a problem within one of your chakras, it may not be enough to just hum or buzz that chakra's note. Our chakras are multidimensional as they are etheric energy. This is a map of the energetic bodies and the harmonics that vibrate them:

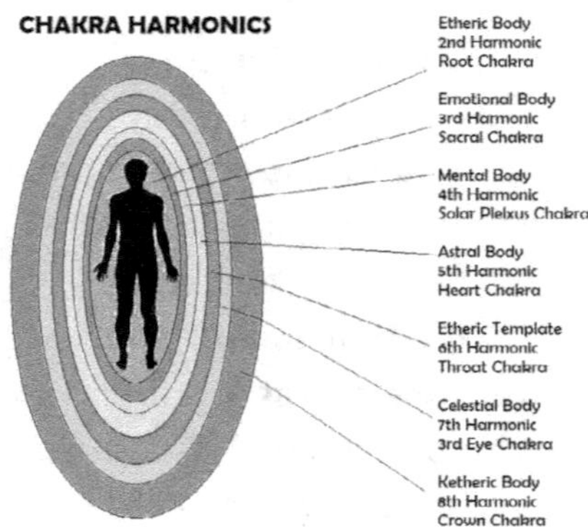

Each of these energetic bodies – Etheric, Emotional, Mental, Astral, and Spiritual – are contained within each chakra. It is possible to work with each of these energetic bodies using the harmonics of the chakra note. If the chakra note is C, its Emotional component is G which is the third harmonic of C. Its Mental component is also the note C except it is an octave higher which is the fourth harmonic. The Astral body, which is out of time and space, interfaces between the physical and spiritual planes. It vibrates to the fifth harmonic of the note C which is E. The Etheric Template level, which is a blueprint of the physical body, resonates with the sixth harmonic of the note C which is G. The seventh harmonic vibrates the Celestial body which is the note B flat. The eighth harmonic is another octave higher C that resonates the Ketheric body which is our energetic "egg" that surrounds all of the energetic levels.

The harmonics will vibrate the chakra's energy field to reset and clear old stuck cellular memory. Here is a chart of the harmonics for each chakra note.

CHAKRA   HARMONICS

8th harmonic	C	C#	D	D#	E	F	F#	G	G#	A	A#	B	Ketheric Body
7th harmonic	A#	B	C	C#	D	D#	E	F	F#	G	G#	A	Celestial Body
6th harmonic	G	G#	A	A#	B	C	C#	D	D#	E	F	F#	Etheric Template
5th harmonic	E	F	F#	G	G#	A	A#	B	C	C#	D	D#	Astral Body
4th harmonic	C	C#	D	D#	E	F	F#	G	G#	A	A#	B	Mental Body
3rd harmonic	G	G#	A	A#	B	C	C#	D	D#	E	F	F#	Emotional Body
2nd harmonic CHAKRA NOTE	C	C#	D	D#	E	F	F#	G	G#	A	A#	B	Etheric Body

If your heart chakra note is E these are its first 8 harmonics

Remember that my understanding is that the chakra energy system is our body's Emotional Energy Distribution System. The chakras connect the entire etheric energy field – this is the energy field that is closest to our physical body and, therefore, closest to our glands, organs, muscles, etc. Humming our chakra notes vibrates these physical areas of our bodies. Most of the time, simply vibrating these areas is sufficient to energize the corresponding chakra. But, if there is an injury in that area of the body that was caused by something not physical, then you will need to understand the harmonics of that chakra to get to the emotional, mental, and spiritual dimensions and the root cause of that issue.

A word of caution, here, is to only work with one chakra's harmonics at a time. These sounds are very powerful.

I learned of this power after a humbling experience. I was proofing the recordings of my harmonic series of notes using choir chimes. After I had been to a recording studio to record each of the possible 12 harmonic series of notes on my chimes, I eagerly awaited to receive the email with the final cuts so that I could try them out. I transferred my chakra harmonics to my mp3 player, and when I went to bed that night, I played the mp3 of the harmonics for each of my chakras. This recording contained the first 16 harmonics of each chakra note. Each of the harmonic series of notes had also been transposed during the recording process to the A = 432 Hz sale. I listened to them all and fell asleep. I was mostly listening for the quality of the sound recording and not for any specific healing purpose.

The next morning, I woke up in quite a funk. I felt really heavy. I was depressed and even briefly considered suicidal thoughts. I was certainly not myself. After a couple of hours, I realized what was going on. I forgot that I had listened to all of those harmonics before falling asleep. Now I knew what to do to get back to normal. I allowed myself to have a cry and release all that energy that was coming up from somewhere unconscious in my energy field. Once that energy was released, I felt MUCH BETTER! There was no way to know after the fact which chakra or chakras had released their old cellular memory. This is why I don't recommend that you work with more than one chakra at a time when you are working with the chakra harmonics.

Chakra Harmonics Meditation

This is a practice for deep work with the Emotional, Mental, and Spiritual dimensions of each chakra.

Using your pitch pipe, play the note of the chakra until you can feel that chakra vibrate. Imagine the feeling of that chakra energy extending out about three inches from your body. Picture that sound moving outwards in concentric circles like when a pebble is tossed into still water. This brings the vibrations into your etheric energy body in the area of your chakra.

Next, while maintaining the feeling of your vibrations three inches or so around your body in the area of that chakra, play the chakra note on the pitch pipe and sing its third harmonic at the same time into the pitch pipe. Do this three or four times until you feel the energy extend out another three inches from your chakra area. If you can't yet feel it, imagine the feeling.

While maintaining the feeling of your vibrations through your Emotional Energy space, play the chakra note on the pitch pipe while humming its fourth harmonic. Feel your vibrations extend out another three inches from your body.

Next, while maintaining the feeling of your vibrations now nine inches from your body, encompassing the etheric, emotional, and mental energy fields, play the chakra note while humming its fifth harmonic. Feel your vibrations extend out to your Astral body now a full foot from your body.

With each higher harmonic imagine or feel the vibrations expanding outwards from your body.

Continue to expand the vibrations out further to the Celestial body by playing the chakra note on the pitch pipe hum its sixth harmonic.

Expand out further by playing the chakra note on the pitch pipe and humming the seventh harmonic.

Finally, imagine expanding out to the edge of your "egg" into the Ketheric body by playing the chakra note on the pitch pipe and humming its eighth harmonic.

Once you have hummed your chakra notes and then connected them through your heart chakra, you have strengthened your Auric field or Biofield. This magnetic energy field around your body is the first line of protection against negative energies. Energizing this auric field helps you maintain your own positive feelings and thoughts while not being as affected by the energies of the outside world. It allows you to stay calmer and more peaceful amidst the energetic chaos that we move through in the world.

To do a really deep dive into a chakra, I have recorded the harmonic series of notes for the first eight harmonics for each chakra with my chimes. These are available on my website for purchase and download. I also offer classes and private sessions online to help you work through these chakra dimensions.

Chapter 16

Harmonics for Systems & Organs

The notes that I used for the aura camera case study were taught to me by Sharry Edwards. Her brilliant work on the emerging science of Human BioAcoustics comes from her love of Mathematics and proclivity for numbers. She also has a very unusual voice that can sing a perfect sine wave. She also has an unusual sense of hearing. She can hear sounds that are coming from people who are ill that the person can't hear. She began by singing back those sounds to people and that made them feel better. Her understanding of the human voice as a biofeedback system for the health and wellness of the body is monumental. She posits that the brain hears the frequencies in the voice as biomarkers for our health and makes adjustments accordingly. Her Note Correlate Chart showcased her understanding of what each note of the scale did both physically and emotionally.

Her work, combined with that of Dorinne Davis, the famous audiologist who discovered the Brain-Ear-Voice connection, inspired me to create horn and voice harmonic recordings that people could listen to and hum along with to raise the frequency of their organs and systems. Dorinne Davis came to her work from the perspective of an audiologist. Sharry Edwards pioneered her work from the perspective of a mathematician. I took both of their perspectives and wove them into my perspective – music. After proving to myself with the aura imaging camera that the harmonics of the notes from Sharry's Note Correlate Chart could really make a difference in my health, I composed several other sound therapy recordings using Sharry's concepts.

Activating Notes: P4, 4+, P5

The Perfect Fourth (P4)

When the distance between two notes is two and a half steps, that interval is called a Perfect Fourth (P4). When two notes that are two and a half steps apart are played together, the most prominent harmonic that you hear is a lower octave of the higher of the two notes. For example, if the two notes are C and F, the most resonant harmonic you hear is F an octave lower. The interval of a P4 creates a low bass sound that pulls energy downward.

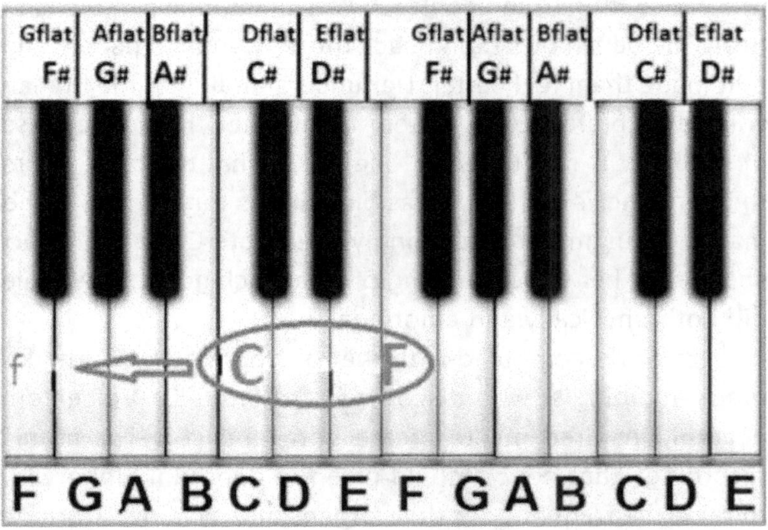

The Augmented Fourth (4+) or Diminished Fifth

This interval is three whole steps apart. It is sometimes called the Tritone (three whole steps) or Devil's interval. Back in the Middle Ages when the monks would sing their chants, this interval was so dissonant that it was considered the Devil's interval and was banned from being used in sacred compositions like the Gregorian Chants and Hymns. This interval creates a very unsettling tension. It begs for resolution back to a harmonious sound. It is usually resolved by subsequently expanding to the next note outward to the P5. The harmonic that is created when this interval is played is a minor third above the low note and a minor third below the upper note. It creates what is known as a diminished chord which is full of tension and pathos.

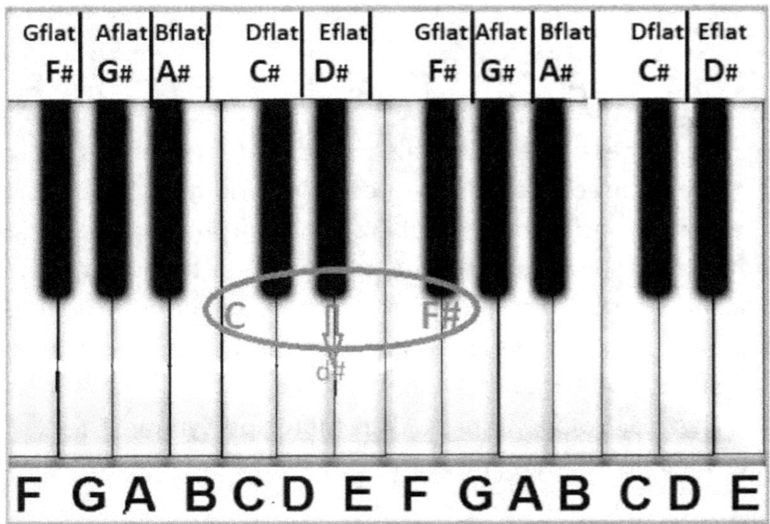

The Perfect Fifth (P5)

When the distance between two notes is three and a half steps apart, that interval is called a Perfect Fifth. When two notes that are three and a half steps apart are played together, the most prominent harmonic that you hear is the octave above the lower of the two notes. For example, if the two notes are C and G, then the most prominent harmonic you will hear is the C an octave higher. This combination of notes moves energy upward.

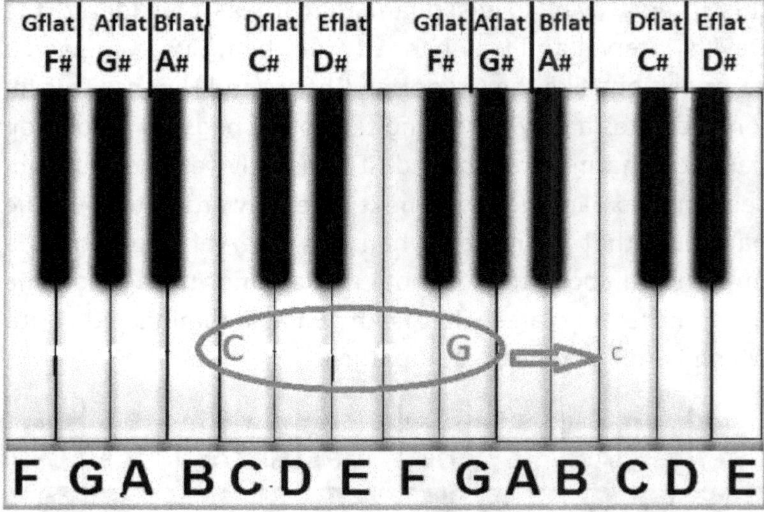

I call these three intervals the *activating* intervals. Playing these three intervals in succession will greatly support the lowest note. The P4 stabilizes and grounds the lowest note, the 4+ creates a balancing tension in the lower note, and the P5 supports the lowest note by giving it structural support. I used these three intervals in my mp3 recordings – Systems and Organs – which are horn and voice harmonics for Thyroid, Colon, Kidneys, Digestion, and Lymph. They are all available at **www.thesoundlady.com**.

Thyroid Support

One of my first mp3 recordings was for raising the frequency of the thyroid. I was diagnosed with underactive thyroid due to Hashimoto's, which is an autoimmune disorder where the immune system attacks the normal thyroid cells. This constant attack fatigues the thyroid and causes it to be under-active. At the time, my symptoms were light, barely notice-able, and the rest of the women in my family also had this disorder and were all taking their prescribed Synthroid med-ication, a synthetic thyroid hormone supplement.

The blood test for this diagnosis measures the amount of Thyroid Stimulating Hormone (TSH) in your body which is pro-duced in the pituitary gland. At the chemical level, thyroid hor-mone T3 converts into T4 which the thyroid uses to keep your metabolism going. Synthroid gives the body more T4 as a sup-plement. Being a person who would rather listen to sounds than take a pill, I decided to compose horn and voice har-monics to energize my thyroid. Listening to these sounds has kept my thyroid working just fine for 15 years. I actually have blood work that shows how listening to these sounds and ton-ing the thyroid notes brought down my TSH level by 7 points.

Now, 15 years later, I continue to work on accessing the root cause of this thyroid issue, and it really seems to have less to do with the amount of T3 and T4 hormones in your system and more to do with the thyroid hormone receptors in your cells. An underactive thyroid produces too much TSH in an attempt to overcompensate for what your hormone re-ceptors are not picking up. The work is to clean up the cells so that receptors can properly function. In my Thyroid Sup-port mp3, I play and sing harmonics on the horn for the notes that correlate to the thyroid. It has helped many people with underactive thyroids.

Kidney Support

Soon after that, I composed another harmonic recording for the kidneys as I had several clients who were having trouble with fluid retention. I warned them not to listen too much or they would be in the bathroom every half hour. This Kidney

Support composition was a major factor in one of my stroke client's recovery. Here is his testimonial:

"I would like to thank Kathleen Nagy for the wonderful support to my Kidney and her use of sound therapy to aid in my Healing. I came to Santa Fe in 2015 after I suffered a Stroke in 2014. The stroke caused my kidneys to be compromised and I have been on Dialysis since 2014. I started using the kidney support audio file created by Kathleen in the summer of 2015...I'm proud to say as of February 15, 2017 my nephrologist has removed me from Dialysis. I stand as a powerful testimony for the Sound Healing support of Kathleen Nagy."

Digestive Support

The Digestive Support mp3 and Colon Support mp3 were composed when my wife was undergoing chemotherapy for breast cancer. The chemo was really throwing off her digestion and elimination. The Digestive Support mp3 contains the harmonics of the organs of digestion and their biological processing – again, from Sharry Edwards' Note Correlation Chart which is Sharry's intellectual property and can be purchased from her website:
https://soundhealthoptions.com/shop/

This harmonic audio file has been very helpful for others who were undergoing chemotherapy as it energized their digestive organs and helped with the nausea that came with the chemotherapy.

The Colon Support mp3 was the result of a case study I did with my wife when her Senna laxative was no longer working. She was in a considerable amount of pain and had a prescription for Oxycontin. When that medication had to be increased, her constipation got out of hand as the Senna was no longer effective.

Below is the note bar graph created by Sharry Edwards' **nVoice** software. This is a type of voice recording software that counts the number of times you use each note of the scale when you speak. Given that Sharry has discovered that each note of the scale has physical and emotional correlations, the software tallies the number of times you use each note when you speak and creates a type of personality trait profile of you based on your speaking pattern of notes.

You can make certain assumptions about the strength of your body's systems and organs based on Sharry's concepts of note correlations to our physical biology. For example, if a note that was hardly ever used in your voice recording correlated to the bladder, I would ask you if you were having incontinence issues since the note was very weak in your voice. Playing that note on a pitch pipe or humming that note gives energy to that frequency so that the brain can use the energy to trigger its self- healing abilities.

Here is a case study using the Colon Support mp3. First, I took my client's voiceprint and analyzed the note bar graph. I saw that notes pertaining to the colon were weak.

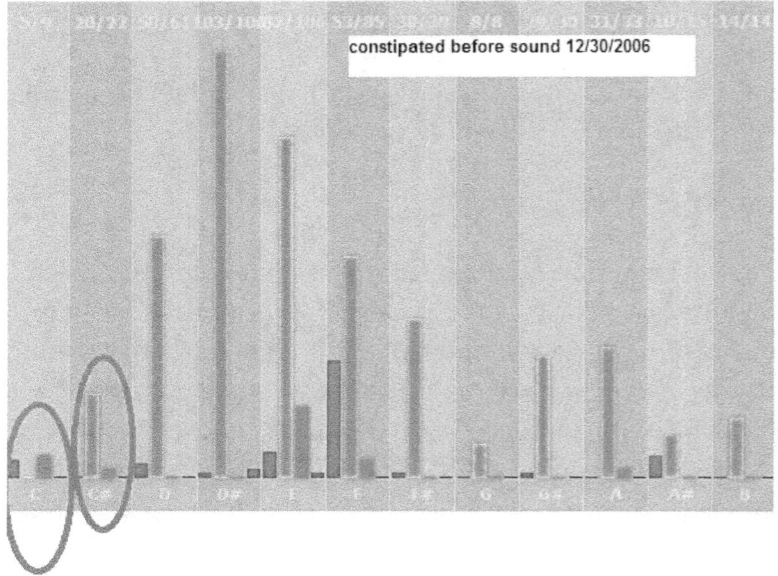

I created a harmonic chord that included those notes and played it for my client for five minutes. We waited ten minutes for those sounds to assimilate into her system, and then I took another voiceprint.

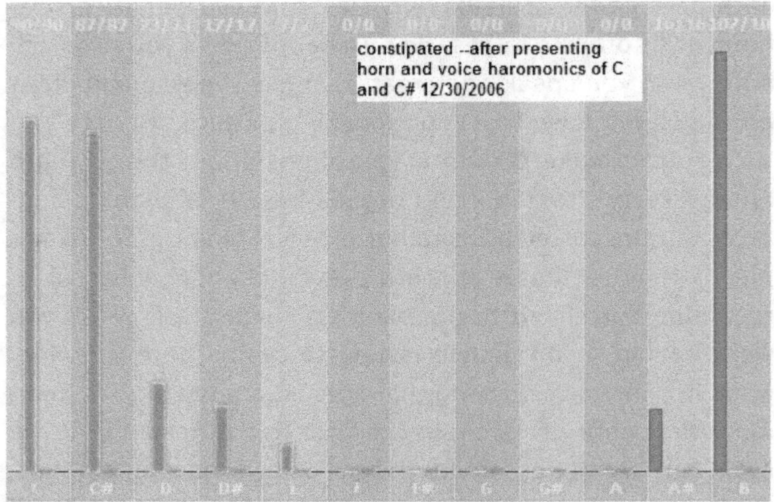

Notice that the notes with initially low energy were now full of energy. After this, a bowel movement was no longer a problem, and she was able to relieve herself within another five minutes.

The same Colon Support mp3 has also helped people with constipation caused by narcotics.

Lymph Support

The last harmonic audio recording that I composed and recorded was for Lymph Support. The Lymphatic system is our body's waste removal system. I created this harmonic for myself when I was trying to expel some parasites that had taken up residence in my head just above the back of the neck. I was out walking my dog in the woods and was swarmed by some black flies. It was the end of May in New

England, and it was prime time for black flies. I had never been bothered by them before, but this swarming was different. I had several bites at the top of my neck, and the next day I had a temperature of 102 and hives all over my body!

The bites were in a spot where, because of the blood-brain barrier, no antibiotics were going to help. I deduced that if I energized the lymph system, I could get them out and be rid of them. I used the notes that governed the body's fluids and created a harmonic composition that would move the lymph more effectively.

Now, when I created this harmonic in 2015, I didn't know that Western medicine was still operating under the consensus that there was no lymph in the brain (they discovered it around 2017). It's a good thing that I didn't know this at the time, otherwise, I might not have tried! After all, I was moving lymph in the brain with harmonics before Western medicine had discovered there WAS lymph in the brain. It turned out to be a very good way to help folks detoxify from all sorts of things, especially heavy metals.

Here's a testimonial from one of my clients, an 80-year-old very health-conscious woman:

"My body is overloaded with heavy metals, especially lead. I'm amazed at the results I have with Kathleen's Lymph Support audio file. It's so powerful that I have to really monitor how frequently I listen to it because of experiencing detox symptoms. I'm so grateful and happy to have an alternative to all the other treatments that I've tried in the past. For me, this is by far the most effective and noninvasive detoxing method."

Chapter 17

Practice & Sound Therapy Tools

Practice – How do you get to Carnegie Hall?

The art of practice is an acquired skill with HUGE benefits. All musicians, artists, and athletes understand the NECESSITY of perfecting their art. You can allot a certain amount of time to practice, but unless you are focused and know *how* to practice, you could be wasting your time. It's hard enough to carve out the time to actually do it, but you also need to develop your practice technique in order to accomplish what you are setting out to accomplish.

Practice is how we learn new things and cement them into our memory. Building new neural pathways takes time and practice. Repeating something over and over can be exceedingly boring and tedious, so you should try to find a technique that incorporates things you love to do. That way, it will not be boring, and you will be more likely to give it a chance to work its magic.

If you think meditating would be a good new skill for you to build, then find a technique that includes doing something you love to do. For many years, I meditated daily while playing harmonics on my French horn. It kept my chops in shape and created complex chords that carried me into meditation. It was a win-win.

For a new sustainable practice of any kind, there must be tangible benefits that are fun to achieve and that will keep you motivated. If you want to start exercising, make it fun for yourself. That way you will be more likely to keep doing it. Some people like the camaraderie of a gym, others enjoy watching DVDs in their own homes.

Learning to meditate is very much the same. Some folks like to meditate in silence, others like to listen to guided meditations, and some people use yoga and breathing as meditation tools. If you can find a way to make it enjoyable, you will more likely incorporate it into your daily life than if it is just another chore for you to perform.

When you do or think something over and over, like repeating a line of a poem to memorize it, you strengthen the pathway in the brain. This process can be likened to a groove in a record album. Those grooves were pressed into the vinyl, and then sound was implanted into them so that the needle would have an accurate way of retrieving the sounds. When a record gets scratched, the needle skips out of the groove and jumps into another path/groove which causes the music to sound out of order. Just like in your brain when a thought, idea, or skill has not been repeated enough to form a strong pathway, your recall of it can be faulty.

Repeating or practicing creates a strong pathway for information to be recalled and performed at will.

The benefits of practice are HUGE. Practice gets results. If you are a goal setter, set a goal. If you are a list maker, make a list of all your practice times so you can cross them off when they're accomplished.

Doing something a little bit every day will make you an expert over time.

What you do today, you will build upon tomorrow and the next day. The neural pathway will get stronger and stronger and be able to hold more and more information. It will become second nature to you. Don't be discouraged if your practice does not yield immediate results. The nature of practice is that it takes time, for it is not an instant gratification process. It will take about a month, for example, for a daily mantra to really settle into your consciousness.

During my undergraduate years at Ithaca College, there were so many hours dedicated to practice. It was and is one of the only music education and applied music colleges where we had to learn to play all of the instruments! Most music schools only require one brass instrument, one woodwind instrument, one stringed instrument, a keyboard, and a percussion class. We had to take a semester each of trumpet, trombone, French horn, tuba, clarinet, flute, saxophone, oboe, bassoon, violin, piano, and percussion.

Practicing each of these instruments over the course of a semester, I learned a lot about efficiency. At first, I expected that two or three times of repeating a difficult section of the music would be enough to cement it into my memory for flawless playback. I found out the hard way that such was not the case. It would frustrate me immensely when I was not able to immediately play the piece perfectly after practicing it for the first time. Over time, I figured out that the time and energy I put into repeating a difficult part of the music over and over and over again for one day's practice session would not yield its fruits until the next day. It always needed to "bake" in my brain overnight. Then, when I would try again the next day, that once difficult and frustrating passage in the music was simple to accurately and consistently perform. Like magic, overnight, all of the finger and eye coordination plus the breathing practice would "gel" so that by morning I had mastered it. The lesson here is that practice does not produce instant gratification. It takes time for the brain to coordinate all the pieces, but if you are patient and persistent, you will reap the benefits of your hard work.

Sound Therapy Tool – French Horn

The best instrument for playing and singing harmonics is the French horn. I understand that most of the folks who will read this book are not French horn players. This section is included for my friends who are French horn players. There are thousands of horn players all over the world who are holding a very powerful instrument in their laps for their own self-healing but don't realize it.

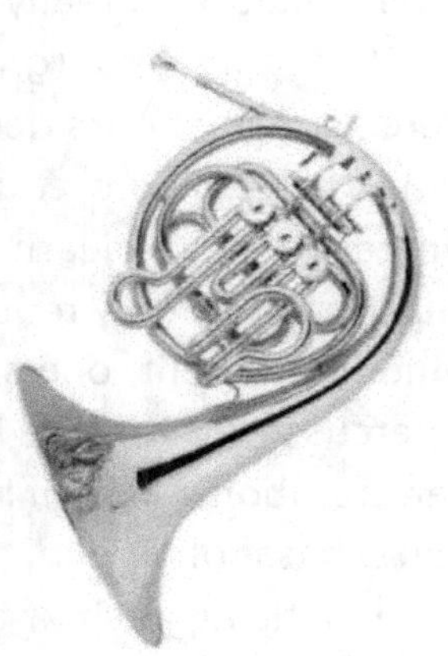

Why is the French horn so good for playing and singing harmonics?

1. It's 144 inches long. That's 12 feet of tubing where the harmonics have a space to expand.
2. It is in the vocal range of most people's singing voices.
3. You hold it in your lap, and you put your hand in the bell which creates a sound energy loop as you blow into it for the sound to go back into your hand and body.

This energy loop is what makes it uniquely qualified as a sound therapy instrument. You are the maker of the sound and the receiver of the sound. You are the transmitter and the receiver with a wide range of pitch possibilities. Personally, I find it easier to play a lower note and sing a higher note. The opposite is possible but depending on the range of the note in your voice, singing the low note and playing a higher note sometimes asks the muscles of the mouth to be tight while the vocal cords are loose. That is harder to do.

When I play my chakra scale on the horn during my meditations, I also hum along at the same time. To receive the maximum vibration, I completely "stop" the sound with my hand and use alternate fingerings a half step below the fingering for the note I want to play, as "stopping" the horn raises its pitch at least a half step. This sends all of the sound from my lips back into my hand and up my arm into my heart. You are now the creator of the sound and the receiver of the sound. You are creating a kind of feedback loop that is exponentially amplifying its effect. This is why I think the French horn is the most powerful sound healing instrument there is.

When I am working on the different dimensions of my root chakra, I place the bell of horn in front of me on both thighs. Blowing the root chakra note sends energy out the bell and into that area of my body. With the horn in this position, I do the Chakra Harmonics Meditation process, *Deep Work with the Emotional, Mental, and Spiritual Dimensions of Each Chakra*. This really helps to feel the energy of the sound going into my body.

If you know your chakra scale notes, you can use your horn to play your body's musical scale which would be very useful for calming the nerves before a performance. Every performance musician has a warmup routine before a concert. Yes, we need to warm up those little lip muscles to get them ready to perform the musical gymnastics required in the written music.

We also need to ready our emotions for the excitement of the performance. Being nervous makes it harder to take deep breathes which are necessary to perform the long phrases in the music. Being nervous causes uneven breathing and a shaky sound. The pressure to play the right note at the right time with the right tuning in balance with the other instruments is enormous. Missing notes too often because of nerves will get you fired. Every orchestral musician knows that there are dozens of other performers waiting to take their chair at the drop of a hat. Performance stress is a very real thing in the classical music industry. There are even prescription drugs that you can take to calm your emotions before performing because many performers cannot tame the nerves no matter how hard they try. If you knew your chakra scale, you could incorporate that into your warmup so that you are in complete control of your chops and your emotions.

Guided Meditation with French Horn

It is normal for a musician who spends hours a day with their instrument to develop a relationship with it. Those who have a relationship of "power with" as opposed to "power over" their instrument have a less stressful and combative performance experience. The horn is a very difficult taskmaster of an instrument. It is difficult to play. You can master it with your will power by making it do what you want it to do which uses an enormous amount of mental energy, or you can work with it, accept its foils, and give yourself the best chance to create a relationship of consensus and cooperation.

Below is a meditation that will help you begin the process of becoming one with your instrument. It is, after all, a piece of metal with specific dimensions and capabilities because of those dimensions. We are human beings; our moods vary from day to day, our needs change from day to day, and our expectations differ from day to day. The horn, however, is a solid piece of unchanging metal.

This meditation for breathing with the horn is a way to create a more equal and inclusive relationship between horn and human. It is a great first step for a warmup routine because, in truth, you don't just have to warm up the lips, you also have to warm up the breath.

Becoming One with Your Instrument

Blow your breath into the horn as you follow its pathway through all the tubing and out the bell.

Imagine your breath going through the mouthpiece and leadpipe into the tuning slides. In your mind, follow the breath out of the tuning slides and into the valves. Visualize your breath going through the tuning slides for each valve. Then follow if out of the valves into and out of the bell and then into your hand.

Once you have the path of your breath through the horn fully visualized, start the process again but this time, add the intention of sending love and gratitude into and through your horn carried on the breath.

Sound Therapy Tool – Pitch Pipe

Pitch Pipe Harmonic Humming

A pitch pipe is like Braille for the ears.

Since it is difficult for most folks to buzz a pitch with their lips and hum another pitch at the same time, I use a pitch pipe first. This helps teach people how to blow a note on the pitch pipe and hum another note at the same time. Blowing a note and humming a note at the same time creates a harmonic chord that the brain will recognize. It creates a similarly pleasant response though it is not as powerful as when you actually make the buzzing with the lips. The pitch pipe is more subtle because there is less lip vibration, but it is nonetheless effective.

For people who have trouble matching a pitch with their voice, humming specific notes is sometimes not possible. This entire book is very much about how to use the energy of your voice to hum specific notes to energize your body. If you can't match a pitch with your voice, these protocols are a nonstarter. But, if you have a pitch pipe, you can blow specific notes and feel their vibrations in your fingertips as well as hear the note in your ears. This practice will begin to reconnect your ear and your voice. Audiologist Dorinne Davis has done wonderful work on this.

What is a Pitch Pipe?

A pitch pipe is a small pipe that sounds tones of standard frequency. Mostly, it is used to establish the starting pitch for voices that sing unaccompanied. The most common type is a circular Free Reed Aerophone. These are discs with the holes for the reeds around the perimeter and with marked openings for each note into which the user blows.

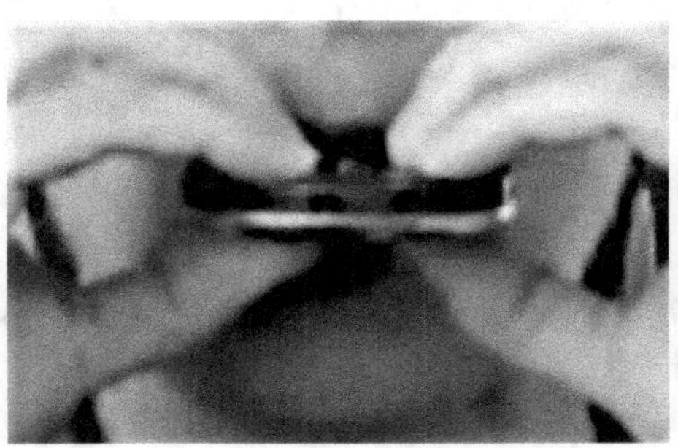

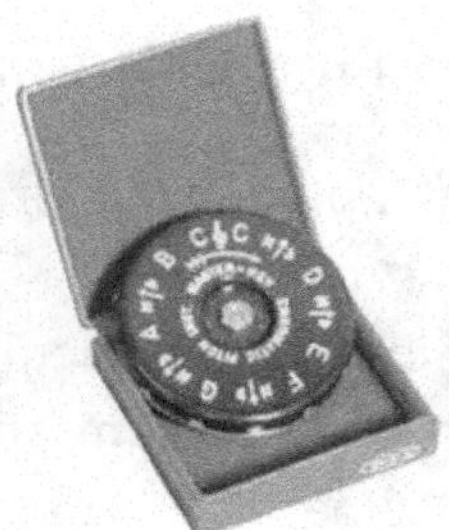

How to Play Harmonics on a Pitch Pipe

Playing harmonics on a pitch pipe will create many of the same harmonics I created with my horn in the aura camera case study. It is the easiest way I know to create predictable harmonics using your voice and a musical instrument **without having to study and play a musical instrument.**

One of the reasons I use a pitch pipe as a sound therapy tool is that you can feel the vibrations of the note that you are blowing with your fingertips. When you blow into it, put all of your fingertips on the top of the pitch pipe and balance it on the bottom with your thumbs. All of the energy meridians in our body – all of our energy pathways – end at our fingertips. This means that not only is your brain able to hear and recognize the harmonic chord you are creating but you can also feel all of the vibrations in your fingertips that are sending the frequencies to all the systems of your body simultaneously.

It's easiest to start with humming the same note that you are blowing into the pitch pipe. The note will wobble around for a while until your voice is perfectly in tune with the pitch pipe. Sometimes it's easier to hum the note an octave above or below the note that you are blowing. Blowing a note on the pitch pipe and humming a note at the same time requires your brain to sort of split in two. Being able to play two notes at the same time that are perfectly in tune with each other will create the harmonic chord. You have to keep adjusting the pitch until you hear the most harmonics.

Take a breath and blow any note on the pitch pipe and hum that same note while you are blowing into the pitch pipe. Do this for 10-15 seconds if possible.

Take a deep breath and blow a low C for 10-15 seconds.

Switch the pitch pipe to a G and blow that note. Try to re-member the sound of it.

Hum the G note to keep its sound in your mind while turning your pitch pipe back to the C note hole.

Hum the G note while blowing the note C into the pitch pipe. Adjust the pitch you are humming until it is perfectly in tune with the C. When you hear the most harmonics, you are per-fectly in tune.

To play the same harmonics and get the same results that I did during my aura camera experiment, follow these steps:

1. Blow into the low C and sing the high C or blow those two holes at the same time.
2. Blow into the low C and sing the B. Do this three times.
3. Blow into the C sharp and sing an A sharp. Do this three times.
4. Blow into the D and sing an A. Do this three times.
5. Blow into the D sharp and sing a G sharp. Do this three times.
6. Blow into the E and sing G. Do this three times.
7. Blow into the F and sing F sharp or blow those two holes at the same time. Do this three times.
8. Then, reverse the notes starting at step #6 working backward through to step #1 so that you end back at the octave of C's. Only play each note once on the reverse.

If this pattern is too difficult, start by just playing the low notes on the pitch pipe while you listen to the Immune

Support mp3 that is available for download at
www.thesoundlady.com.

Sound Therapy Tool – Plastic Corrugated Tube

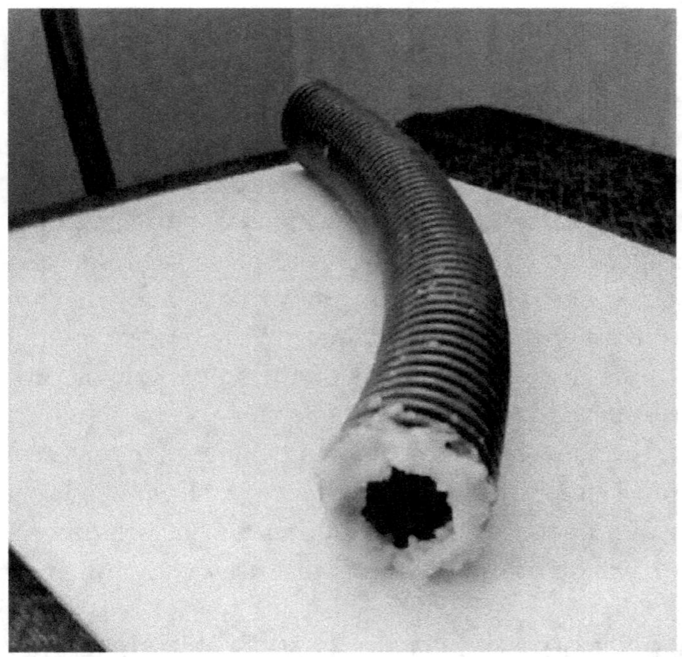

This is something that I made to help me vibrate parts of my
body from the outside with my voice which is different from
humming and vibrating your body from the inside with your
voice. You can get this type of plastic tubing at any hardware
store in the gardening department. You can get it cut to any
length. To start, I would suggest that you get three feet of
tubing and cut it into a one-foot piece and a two-foot piece.
Melt some candle wax and dip one of the ends into the wax
to coat the jagged edge of the plastic pipe. This will protect
your lips from being cut on the plastic.

You can use this tubing to blow into, buzz into, and sing
harmonics into while you place it on the part of your body

that you are working on. The warmth of your breath is an immediate comfort that relaxes the part of the body you are working with. The different lengths can accommodate different areas of your body. You can use the one-foot tube to sing into your thyroid, lungs, or shoulder, for example, and the two-foot tube can be used for hips or knees (if you are sitting down).

You can use a full three-foot length of tubing to work on your Root and Sacral chakras if you are doing the Chakra Harmonics Meditation process in **Deep Work with the Emotional**, **Mental, and Spiritual Dimensions of Each Chakra**. Hum into one end of the tube and place the other end on the chakra center either in front of your body or on your spine. Each chakra has an opening in the front of our bodies and in the back of our bodies on the spinal column. Experiment with both to really feel the energy of the sound going into your body. I don't recommend longer than three feet of tubing. This is too long of a distance to fill with your breath and sound and be felt at the other end of the tube. Your breath will be cold when it hits the other end of the tube.

Sound Therapy Tool – Crystal Healing Bowls

I used crystal healing bowls for my own meditations early in my sound healing endeavors. I would play and sustain the pitch of the bowl while I sang the harmonics of that pitch into the bowl. It was a great way to get my head into the vibrations. These are a favorite instrument for sound bath concerts. The bowls come in a wide range of frequencies and they have a very resonant and expansive sound that is easily felt in the body.

I had trouble with two such sound bath concerts that I attended. The musicians intended for their sounds to wash over and soothe the audience. As they played, they improvised on keyboards, crystal bowls, and bass guitar while using intuition to guide what notes to play. At times, this created great dissonances that made me feel nauseous, and I had to leave the concert. I am sensitive to sound for sure, but I bet I'm not the only one who has had this reaction to a sound bath concert.

Being subjected to powerful resonant sounds that you do not need can give you a headache, make you feel anxious, nauseous, or agitated. For this reason, I offer sessions and classes for you to discover your personal chakra scale which is the musical key of your body. I provide you with music to hum along with that is in your body's key. My recordings create a sound bath that is personal and customized to your body's musical key. This will ground, center, and calm you. Your body is so happy to hear its own song that it responds instantly with joy and peace which raises your overall frequency state of being.

The drawback of crystal healing bowls for me is that they only play one pitch per bowl, and one person can only play two bowls at a time. They can get expensive and hard to transport. To overcome these obstacles, I graduated to Choir Chimes.

Sound Therapy Tool – Choir Chimes

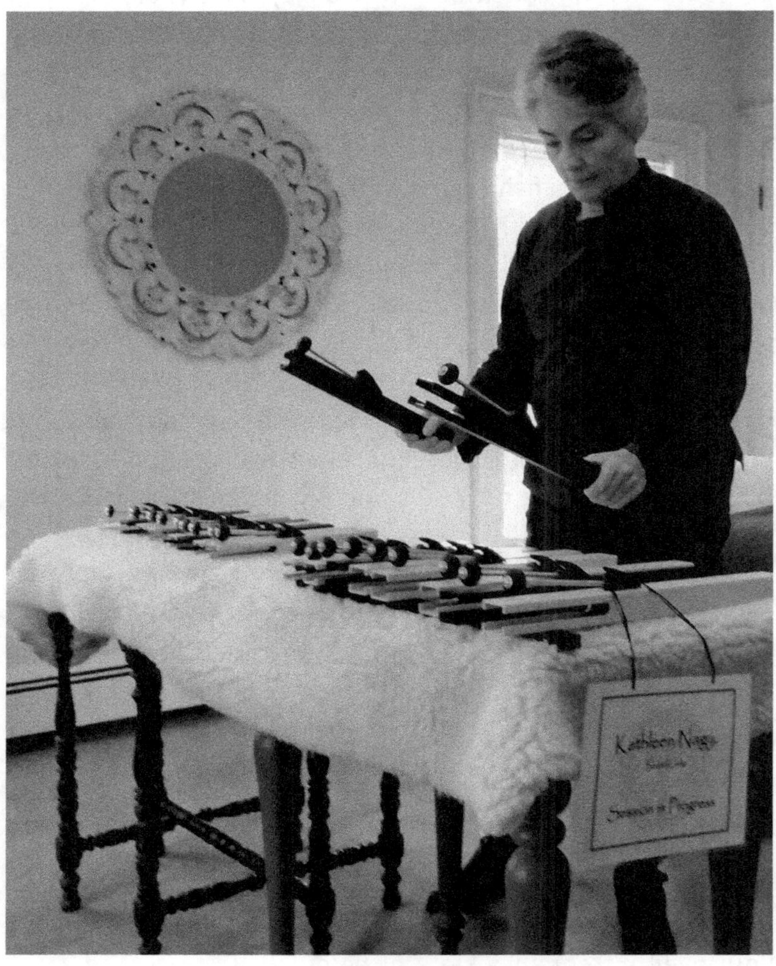

I **LOVE** these chimes. They are made by Malmark. I have four octaves of them. These are the new age edition of handbells. If you have ever played in or listened to a handbell choir, these are similar but better. Handbells sound very bright, and due to their bell curves and wide-open ends, their harmonics are not as organized as in the Choir Chimes. The Choir Chimes have a much darker sound that is richer and full of harmonics due to their elongated and hollow shape. The harmonics have a chance to sound in these tubes much more than in handbells. Harmonics and full-spectrum sound are more useful for sound therapy than a bell or a gong for creating specific harmonic patterns. These are the chimes that I use to record all of the chakra chimes scales and guided meditation mp3s for **Your Personal Chakra Scale** sessions.

Chapter 18

Voice Analysis Software

Sharry Edwards has created hundreds of software templates where the client's stressed frequencies are compared to the frequency biomarkers for all kinds of diseases and ailments. These software templates identify very specific and accurate frequencies like 27.34 Hz. These types of software templates require a certification of training to use, but there is another type of software that Sharry has created called *nanoVoice,* a micro-version of *nVoice*. This software doesn't require a certificate of training to own and operate. It is not as specific as the other templates. Instead of identifying specific frequencies, it counts how many times you use each note when you speak. It identifies your musical speaking pattern. You record your voice using any microphone as opposed to the other templates that require a special microphone. When you finish recording, you receive a graph that shows how many times you used each note as you spoke.

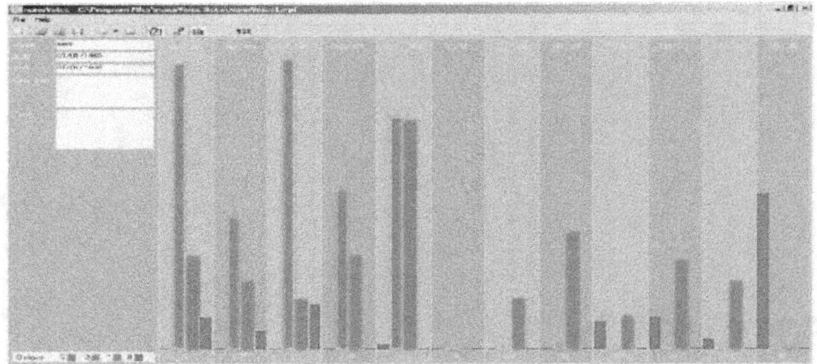

This shows your notes that have weak energy and notes that have too much energy compared to the rest of your vocal pattern. Sharry has devised an ingenious way of correlating each note of the scale with emotional and physical properties. When you purchase this inexpensive software you will receive several charts with physical and emotional note correlations. By comparing your weak energy notes with the note correlate chart, you can easily see which notes you need to strengthen that relate to your weakness. Then you can use your pitch pipe to play and hum these notes to give them energy. The best part is that you can do before and after voice prints which will verify whether or not what you are doing is working.

Record your voice into the software.

Identify which notes and body systems need more energy.

Play those notes on a pitch pipe or hum them for about five minutes.

Wait ten minutes for the sounds to assimilate into your system. Record another voiceprint to see if those notes now have more energy.

This is a fabulous way to check your work. It gives you proof that what you are doing is helping.

You have seen one example of this kind of session in Chapter 16 regarding a weak colon. Here is another case study in which the initial voiceprint recording showed a weakness in the note B.

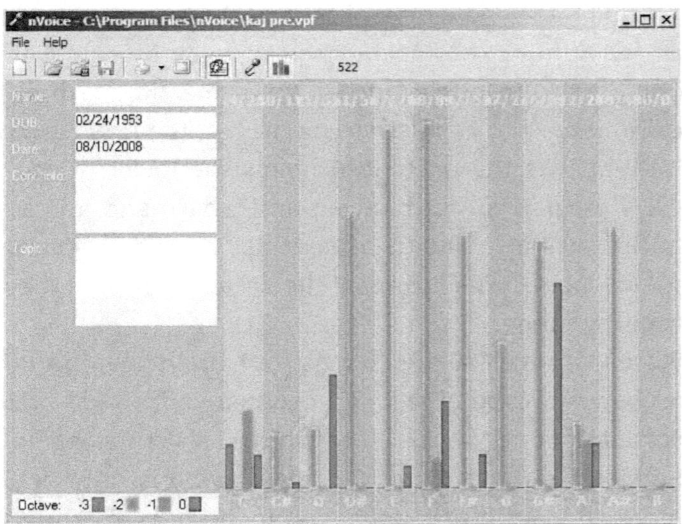

After humming and playing B on the pitch pipe for about three minutes, this was the result:

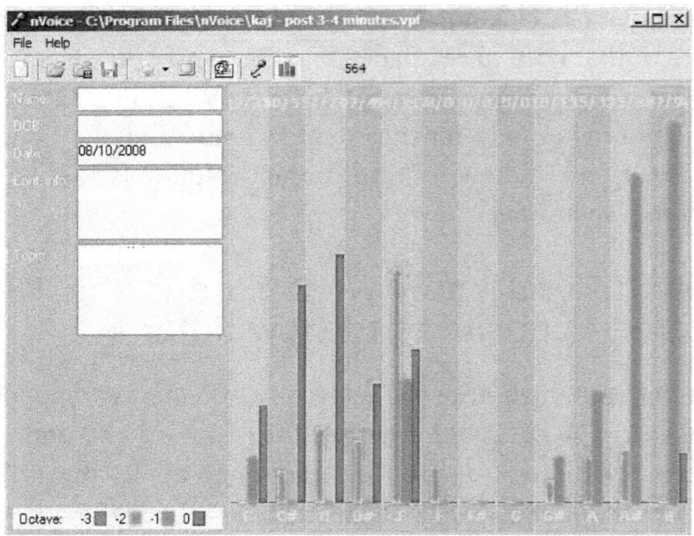

Notice that the B is now high in energy. Also notice that the F, F sharp, and G which were in the normal range in the initial graph are now low in energy in the second graph. Those notes can now be energized by humming and playing the G and F sharp note on a pitch pipe. When two low energy notes are right next to each other, you can blow into those two holes on the pitch pipe at the same time. When two notes right next to each other are played, the first harmonic you will hear is the note right below the lower of the two notes. This means that blowing an F sharp and a G at the same time will also energize the note F. Another voiceprint could now be recorded to see if the notes are now in the normal energy range.

According to Sharry Edwards, our brain's wiring determines how we respond to and process sounds. A left-brained person, someone who is very logical, will process sound 180-degrees differently from a person who is right-brained or very creative. That means that if the note G is missing from the voice print, some people will want more of the note G and some people will want the note C sharp instead. When a frequency is lacking, a left-brained person wants to hear more of that note to rebalance that frequency. In contrast, a right-brained person wants to hear the opposite note of a weak energy note to balance the low energy note.

Figuring out the left or right brain solution is easy – just play the weak note.

How do you know what note is the 180-degree opposite of the low note?

Imagine that the C note is the low or weak energy frequency. The note C = 16.35 Hz. Multiply that note by 180 and you have 2,943. Then, divide that frequency by 2's down into the same octave as the 16.35 Hz C note and you get 22.99 Hz. This is equal to the note F sharp.

Let's use an A note for another more familiar example. The orchestras of the world all tune to an A which equals 440 Hz. If you multiply 440 Hz by 180, you get 79,200. Then, if you divide that number by 2's down into the same octave as 440, you will get 618.75 which is the note D sharp. The octave of the A note would start at 440 Hz and go up to 880 Hz. Right in the middle of those two notes is 618.75 Hz. The note D sharp is the mathematic and geometric opposite of the note A, 440 Hz.

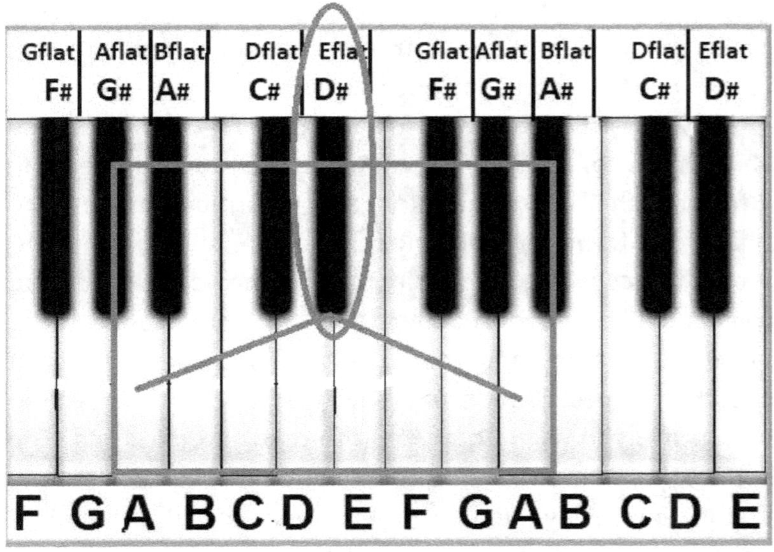

In terms of sound versus math, as you move up the A scale, away from the A note, D sharp is harmonically the furthest away from the note A in terms of resonance. The next note after D sharp is E. It is the perfect fifth of the A note, the most mathematically coherent with A other than an octave A.

The opposite note creates tension. The tension is useful for holding the lower note in the proper balance. For instance, if you want to balance a note that has too much energy – perhaps that note correlates to an overtightened muscle – you would play the opposite note to rebalance and relax that muscle. When you purchase the ***nanoVoice*** application from Sharry Edwards, you get a manual that explains all of this in great detail.

As you practice with this, know that when you are comparing before and after voice prints, you **MUST** talk about the same topic that you talked about when you were recording the first voiceprint. Where attention goes, energy follows. Repeating the same topic while talking and recording the second voiceprint is crucial.

BioAcoustic Research Associates use an excerpt from the children's book, *The Velveteen Rabbit* to read from. Reading it for both the before and after voice recording ensures continuity of information. Obviously, if you are talking about different topics when you are recording the voiceprints, you will get a different vocal pattern of notes. For instance, if you talked about something that upset you in the first voiceprint and then talked about something you loved in the second voiceprint, you would get very different note patterns. The sound of our voice differs depending on what we are talking about. This is a valuable tool for doing sound energy balancing that proves the efficacy of the session.

Chapter 19

Online Courses & Sessions

At **www.thesoundlady.com** you can join a scheduled class or sign up for a private session. You can also download a Do-It-Yourself instructional video. The course information is available in these three formats to accommodate people with different learning preferences. The only course that is not available for class or DIY format is **Your Personal Harmonic Clearing** as it would be too detailed and varied for that format. The three courses that are offered online are:

Your Personal Chakra Scale/ Your Body's Musical Key
Immune Support Harmonic Humming
Your Personal Harmonic Chakra Clearing

Your Personal Chakra Scale/ Your Body's Musical Key

This is a three-hour Live online class given by me, The Sound Lady, Kathleen Nagy. Here we highlight that your chakras are the hardware your body uses to distribute your emotions into your cells. **The sound spectrum of our individual voices reveals the musical key to which our body's emotions are tuned.** Learning your body's personal chakra scale notes and your body's musical key will balance your emotions and calm your nerves for relief of Anxiety, PTSD, Insomnia, and Depression. You will gain first-hand experience of your chakras actually vibrating. The subtle vibration helps to release stuck cellular emotional memory from the cells of your body that could be causing you pain and sleepless nights.

Included in this course is a simple humming technique using notes that were derived from the sound of your sigh and your personal vocal range. This humming technique can unlock emotional cellular memory AND release unconscious feelings that are stuck and no longer serving you.

In this three-hour online class, you will discover:
*How to hum your personal chakra scale and feel your chakras vibrate in your body
*How to use your chakra notes to relieve emotionally triggered pain in all parts of the body
*How to teach your clients to do this for themselves

Also included with this course (mp3s):
*Your Personal Chakra Scale Guided Meditation
*Your Personal Chakra Scale without the guided meditation
*Connecting Your Chakras Through the Heart

Immune Support Harmonic Humming

This two-hour online course is for body and energy workers who want to add another tool to their healing toolboxes.

In this course you will learn:
*How humming can increase a coronavirus killing molecule called Nitric Oxide

*How to hum to increase Nitric Oxide in nasal passages and sinuses

*How to create harmonics with your voice using tongue positions and vowel sounds

*The importance of the third harmonic to the structural integrity of a weak note

*How to buzz with your lips for health benefits similar to yoga exercises

*How to play a pitch pipe in lieu of humming

*How to play harmonics on a pitch pipe

*How to play the same immune-boosting series of harmonic chords that were used in my aura imaging case study

Also Included with this course:
*Immune Support mp3

Your Personal Harmonic Chakra Clearing (Private Session)

Once you have scheduled and completed Level 1 of "Your Personal Chakra Session" with me, this is Level 2. Humming your chakra notes vibrates the physical body in the area of the chakra. In many cases, this is sufficient to reset the chakras balance and energy. Sometimes you need to go deeper. You may find that you need extra work on some of your chakras that simple humming of their notes doesn't address. Learn to hum the notes that correspond to your chakra's emotional, mental, and spiritual dimensions.

Included in this session:
*First 16 harmonics chimed for each of your chakras (mp3 recordings)
*A recording of your zoom video session

Your Personal Harmonic Chakra Clearing (Online class)

This 8-week online class includes everything from Your Personal Chakra Scale class to how to play the harmonics that correlate to each chakra's emotional, mental, and spiritual dimensions. The first week is how to hum your personal chakra scale and how to connect your chakras through the heart. The next seven weeks will be a deep dive into each chakra starting from the root. You will learn to play the harmonics that correlate to the emotional, mental, and spiritual dimensions of each chakra. You will spend a week working with these sounds for each chakra which will give you time to process anything that comes up to be cleared. Working this way from the Root to the Crown over a period of about two months offers a complete clearing that will last. It makes sense to start at the Root and build support and balance from the bottom to the top.

This class includes (mp3s):
*Your Personal Chakra Scale Guided Meditation
*Your Personal Chakra Scale without the guided meditation
*Connecting Your Chakras Through the Heart
*Chimes recording of the first 16 harmonics of each of your seven major chakras

About the Author

Kathleen is a lifelong musician. After majoring in Music Education and Applied Music on French horn at Ithaca College, she did graduate work at Yale University in French horn and Orchestral Conducting. This led her to decades of experience teaching choral and instrumental music classes in public and private schools from elementary through adult education. In that time, she also directed many musical theater productions with high school and college students.

After 20 years of performing in symphony orchestras, Kathleen spent the last couple of decades as a BioAcoustic Research Associate specializing in Voice Energy Analysis and Acoustic Biofeedback for sports or muscle injuries. She was a member of the Board of Directors for Sound Health International of Ohio for 4 years (2005-2009) and worked closely with Sharry Edwards, the founder of Human BioAcoustics.

Now, at the culmination of her life's work, having foraged through the ingredients of crafted "classical" melody, harmony, and structure to find the power, beauty, and healing properties of tone and harmonics, she specializes in teaching you how to hum the sounds that are good for your body. She composed most of the music for her French horn solo CD, *Prayer Songs*, which is available along with Kathleen's other sound healing products and services.

Find out for yourself at **www.thesoundlady.com**!

www.ingramcontent.com/pod-product-compliance
Lightning Source LLC
Chambersburg PA
CBHW071421150726

48000CB00001B/434